The
ANTIBIOTIC
ALTERNATIVE

The Natural Guide to
Fighting Infection and Maintaining
a Healthy Immune System

Cindy L. A. Jones, PH.D.

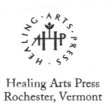

Healing Arts Press
Rochester, Vermont

Healing Arts Press
One Park Street
Rochester, Vermont 05767
www.InnerTraditions.com

Healing Arts Press is a division of Inner Traditions International

*Note to the reader: This book is intended as an informational guide. The remedies,
approaches, and techniques described herein are meant to supplement, and not to be a
substitute for, professional medical care or treatment. They should not be used to treat
a serious ailment without prior consultation with a qualified health care professional.*

Library of Congress Cataloging-in-Publication Data

Jones, Cindy L. A., 1956-
    The antibiotic alternative : the natural guide to fighting infection and
    maintaining a healthy immune system / Cindy L. A. Jones.
        p. cm.
    Includes bibliographical references and index.
    ISBN 0-89281-877-8 (alk. paper)
        1. Communicable diseases—Alternative treatment. 2. Antibiotics—
    Side effects. 3. Drug resistance in microorganisms. 4. Naturopathy.
    5. Herbs—Therapeutic use. I. Title.

RC112 .J66 2000
616.9'046—dc21

                                                            00-039574

Printed and bound in Canada

10 9 8 7 6 5 4 3 2 1

Text design and layout by Rachel Goldenberg
This book was typeset in Caslon with Copperplate as the display typeface

The
ANTIBIOTIC
ALTERNATIVE

CONTENTS

1 MEDICAL MICROBIOLOGY

WHAT ARE PATHOGENS?

Pathogens, which we sometimes call germs, are actually a variety of microorganisms that are at the root of disease. The word *microbes* refers to tiny organisms that cannot be seen without the aid of a microscope. The first of them were seen by the Dutch naturalist Antonie van Leeuwenhoek in 1675. Antonie van Leeuwenhoek was an amateur microscope builder who saw a previously unseen world when he looked through a microscope at a droplet of water. In this drop of water he viewed a world of tiny living things that he called "wee animalcules," for "tiny animals." We now call these tiny living things microorganisms, or microbes for short. These life-forms are 1–2 micrometers in size, fifty times smaller than anything the unaided human eye can see.

These microorganisms can belong to any of the five kingdoms of living things: Monera, Protista, and Fungi as well as the more familiar Plant and Animal kingdoms. Living things in these categories are subdivided down to the genus and species level in a method of naming things that was outlined in the eighteenth century by the Swedish botanist Carolus Linnaeus. It was a shorthand designation for the cumbersome naming system that was in vogue at the time. Just as all plants are denoted using this so-called binomial system of genus name followed by species name, so too are microorganisms.

Microbes can be either beneficial or detrimental to humans, depending on their food source. Microbes are a necessary part of the food web in their role as decomposers, recycling organic matter. Other microbes live in the intestines of human beings and animals to aid digestion and nutrient absorption.

WHERE DID THOSE PESKY BACTERIA COME FROM?

Chances are that bacteria were the first form of life on earth, even older than humans, even older than the dinosaurs. Early life on planet Earth probably arose from simple chemicals plus energy, a process referred to as chemical evolution. The Russian biochemist A. I. Oparin suggested this hypothesis as early as 1922, but it was not tested until the 1950s, when Stanley Miller combined the simple chemicals of hydrogen gas, ammonia, methane, and water vapor with energy in the form of heat and electricity. From these simple conditions that may have mimicked early times on Earth, organic compounds, including amino acids and nucleic acids, were formed. In a sense, in Earth's early history, lakes may have served as an organic soup for dissolving the chemicals necessary for the evolution of chemicals into life.[1]

From these small organic building blocks, it is conceivable that aggregates formed and reacted with each other, building more-complex molecules. For instance, the nucleic acids combined to form DNA, amino acids reacted to form proteins, and sugars reacted to form carbohydrates. Small droplets of these molecules could have been bound together in some way to make a cell-like structure that evolved further to create the first living thing, a bacterium. In another two billion years, these bacteria could have evolved into the more-complex cells (eukaryotic cells) that make up more-complex organisms.

These single-celled organisms belong to the kingdom Prokary-
ote, also referred to as Monera. Bacteria are divided into
gram-positive and gram-negative groups, based on whether they can
be stained with a violet-colored dye. This ability is due to differences in the architecture of the cell wall and is important in terms of
the action of antibiotics. The cell wall is a rigid structure surrounding the cell membrane, giving the bacteria its shape. Bacteria are
also identified by their shapes—round or cocci, rod or bacilli, and
spiral or spirilla.

Bacteria are adaptable to their environment. One reason is that
they grow very quickly, sometimes dividing once every thirty minutes, making one become two. At this rate, in one hour there would
be two bacteria, and, more dramatically, in just ten hours there would
be 1,048,576 of these organisms. This high rate of reproduction
makes bacteria more prone to genetic mutations. Thus, pressure from
their surroundings may allow new forms of the bacteria to grow that
are better adapted to the environment. This is how antibiotic resistance occurs. Although different kinds of bacteria can survive
extremes of temperature, most common bacteria can be killed by
heat. This is why many foods are cooked and one way that we ster-
ilize things. Bacterial growth can also be slowed by cold, which is
the reason we refrigerate food.

FUNGI

Fungi differ from bacteria in that they are eukaryotic, a more complex cell type with a visible nucleus. Most fungi consist of more than
one cell and have hyphae (the threadlike filaments that make up the
mycelium of a fungus) rather than roots, as plants do. Mushrooms
are the reproductive part of some types of fungi that reproduce by
forming spores. These spores can withstand extremes in the environment, such as heat, cold, and drying. This is one reason that fungal infections can be so persistent. The initial disease will go away,
but at a later time the spores germinate and cause the infection to
recur. There are also single-celled fungi, like the yeasts, that divide
in a manner similar to that of bacteria.

VIRUSES

Viruses are of a different sort, not even considered a living organism by most scientists. They are not cells but are more like a particle that contains a piece of either DNA or RNA. This core is surrounded by a coat, usually made of protein. Alone, viruses are inert and require a host cell even to reproduce. Once a virus attaches to and enters a cell, it can control the proteins made by the cell. By forcing the cell to make proteins necessary for viral reproduction, the virus replicates to very high numbers until the cell bursts open, releasing millions of viral particles. Treatments for viral diseases are aimed at blocking the ability of the virus to make new DNA or RNA once inside the host cell. Examples of viral diseases are colds, flu, measles, mumps, and some types of meningitis.

Because viruses cannot be seen by normal light microscopes, they were identified much later than bacteria were. In fact, noting that infectious agents could pass through a filter that would hold back bacteria led scientists to suspect that an even smaller pathogen existed. In 1898 foot-and-mouth disease was the first disease identified as being caused by an infectious agent smaller than a bacterium, but it wasn't until the electron microscope came into use in the 1930s that viruses were actually identified and seen. Before this time, they were considered to be fluid rather than particulate. Although there are many identified viruses today, there is no classification system for them such as the one used for bacteria and fungi.

Most human beings have inactive, or latent, viruses in the body. These viruses remain harmless until an opportunity arises to cause infection—for instance, when the human body is compromised in some way, when the immune system is not on its toes, when stress is acting on the body. Viruses can also cause some types of cancer. Liver cancer, cervical cancer, and some leukemias are caused by viruses. These specific viruses interact with the human cellular DNA in a way that creates new proteins. In this case, the new proteins do not act just for the viruses' survival, but cause uncontrolled growth in the human cell as well. This uncontrolled growth is cancer. There may also be other ways in which viruses affect our bodies that we are not aware of yet.

PROTOZOA

Protozoa are single-cell eukaryotic parasitic organisms that are part of the kingdom Protista. Most protozoa do not cause disease, but some can bring about dysentery and intestinal infections. You have probably heard of "Montezuma's revenge," a diarrhea produced by a protozoan called *Giardia lamblia* as well as by other organisms. This organism is present in fouled water, one reason that water one drinks in the wild needs to be purified in some way.

WHAT CAUSES INFECTIOUS DISEASE?

The word *infection* actually means "pus." It was given this name owing to the large amounts of pus associated with it. As early as the period of the Roman Empire, scientists suggested that disease was caused by tiny, invisible, airborne seeds that could be breathed into the body. But it was the French microbiologist Louis Pasteur, in the late 1800s, who made the connection between microbes and disease and developed what we call the germ theory of disease. At that time, most people thought that bacteria arose spontaneously from dead materials and thus caused putrefaction. Pasteur, however, proved that bacteria were present in the air and then permeated foods to cause putrefaction. Pasteur showed that microorganisms, such as the spores from mold that were found in spoiled food, could be filtered from the air. He then demonstrated that heat could kill many of these microorganisms. Using this knowledge, he performed the most convincing experiment. Putting a nutrient liquid into a flask, he melted the opening of the flask into a series of curves. This allowed air to enter the flask, but not microorganisms. Microorganisms, being basically immobile, could not move through the curves as the air did. He then heated the liquid to boiling, which would kill any microorganisms already present in the liquid. After cooling, he noted that the flask could remain this way for eighteen months without becoming spoiled or putrefied, proving that spores did not arise spontaneously from the liquid. With this information, he also discovered a method for removing microbes from milk, thus eliminating the spread of tuberculosis and typhoid through milk. Gradually, people became convinced that life had to arise from life rather than spontaneously.[2]

The German bacteriologist Robert Koch further advanced the germ theory of disease in the late nineteenth century to one germ/one disease. He was a frustrated physician who realized that he could not cure a disease when he did not know its cause. Koch showed that anthrax in sheep and tuberculosis were both related to the presence of specific bacteria. He outlined four requirements to determine whether a given microbe causes a specific disease. These requirements are known as Koch's postulates:[3]

1. A specific organism must be present in all cases of the disease.
2. The organisms must be able to be isolated and grown in the laboratory.
3. The isolated organism must cause the same disease when injected into another animal.
4. The same organism must be able to be isolated from the second animal and grown in culture.

These criteria have been essential for determining the agents that cause infectious disease, beginning with tuberculosis and cholera.

Even though we are in constant contact with infectious microbes, infectious disease is quite rare. This brings up a second theory about the cause of disease. A Russian scientist of the same era as Pasteur, Élie Metchnikoff, observed that white blood cells have the ability to engulf bacteria.[4] This finding led him to believe that white blood cells protect the body from infection and thus that infections are the result of a weak host. At the time, the idea of one cell "eating" another was too much for people to comprehend, and his theory was not accepted until much later. Ultimately, however, his work became the foundation for the field of immunology.[5]

Today it is generally accepted that infectious disease is a result of a combination of bacterial pathogens and a weakened immune system. Although individuals with a strong immune system probably are better able to resist disease, given an injection of anthrax bacteria they will nonetheless succumb to the disease. Infection was the most common cause of disease up to the twentieth century, the main ones being tuberculosis, syphilis, diphtheria, plague, meningitis, malaria, pneumonia, and infections as the result of childbirth.

HOW DID INFECTIOUS DISEASE BEGIN?

During the course of human existence, we have seen the coming and going of many different infectious diseases. It was probably the agricultural revolution that first brought about infectious disease. The increased numbers of population centers that were born when we evolved from hunter-gatherers to farmers put people in much closer contact with each other as well as with animals. Animal diseases adapted themselves to humans and fouled both water and land. Rodents and mosquitoes soon learned to coexist with humans, and also spread disease. Diets were centered on very few foods, possibly leading to nutritional deficiencies that didn't help boost immunity.[6]

Epidemics, common during the second century, are said by some historians to have brought down the Roman Empire. Among these epidemics were smallpox and measles. The bubonic plague, or black death, devastated civilizations during the sixth and seventh centuries. But the plague's most memorable appearance began around 1300 A.D. in Asia and spread westward through Europe. During the 1600s the bubonic plague flourished in Spain, and its effects didn't end until about 1800. The bubonic plague is caused by a bacterium called *Yersinea pestis*, which is carried by fleas. The bacteria enter the host when the flea bites and take up residence in the lymph glands. Here they cause the characteristic swelling of the armpit, groin, or neck, depending on which lymph gland becomes infected. This form of the disease typically caused death in 60 percent of its victims.[7]

Because of poor living conditions in European cities during the time of the plagues, diseases flourished. Neither bathing nor changing clothes was common, so human bodies were ideal hosts for fleas and lice. Lack of sewers put both human and animal wastes on the streets. Drinking water was not purified, as it is today, and often carried disease. Any person who lived through that time had to have a good immune system. The explorers who traveled to the New World were undoubtedly immunologically strong, but most likely were also carriers of the European diseases. When they came into contact with native people who had never before been exposed to the diseases of other continents, the native people contracted the diseases. In fact, much of the native populations of Mexico and Central America were killed by smallpox and typhus, brought to their countries by the Spanish explorers.[8]

Something similar happened when the European-Americans brought African slaves to the New World. With these slaves came additional diseases, such as malaria, which also killed Native Americans. Over time, however, native populations were able to build immunity and increase in population, at least in Mexico and South America. Yellow fever and cholera were new diseases of the seventeenth century, possibly of African origin. There are still epidemics in modern times. The first was the influenza pandemic in 1918, which killed twenty-five to thirty million people, more than were killed during all of World War I. This was followed by an epidemic of encephalitis, an infection of the brain and spinal cord, and another deadly influenza epidemic in 1920. Cholera is still seen today with new strains emerging.[9]

Infectious disease is the leading cause of death worldwide; in the United States it ranks third (up from fifth a few years ago).[10] Infectious diseases have been replaced by diseases that better reflect our modern lifestyle—such chronic degenerative conditions as lung cancer and heart disease. Why? Nobody can say for sure, but theories abound. Reasons given range from the use of vaccinations and antibiotics to a constitutional change in the human being. We will discuss the role antibiotics and vaccinations may or may not have played in the decline of major infectious diseases in chapter 3. Among other changes that have transpired in the past one hundred years, during the decline of infectious diseases, new foods and better ways of storing those foods have come into use. This improved nutrition may contribute to strengthened resistance in people. Dramatic improvements in waste control, such as sewers, as well as the availability of clean water, at least in developed nations, may also have played a part.

Another theory about the decline in infectious disease is pathogens themselves have undergone changes. Bacteria and viruses have one major goal, and that is survival. If they are potent enough to kill their host, they also lose by no longer having a host. If they transform themselves enough to still benefit from the host without killing it, they win by having a larger pool of hosts. In this way, evolutionary pressure on the pathogens themselves may have forced mutations, allowing host and pathogen to live in closer harmony. Some microbiologists believe that when the common cold first came into existence, it was a deadly killer. With time it evolved into just a major inconvenience.

MAJOR INFECTIOUS DISEASES

Let us take a look at some of the current major infectious disease killers.

TUBERCULOSIS

Tuberculosis, also called consumption or white plague, is one of the oldest diseases known. As long ago as the mid-fourteenth century B.C., it took the life of King Tutankhamen, the Egyptian pharaoh. It has also been found in the bones of the mummified remains of lesser known Egyptians.[11] The disease primarily affects the lungs and then kills slowly. The causative microorganism, *Mycobacterium tuberculosis,* was one of the many organisms discovered by Robert Koch in 1882.

In 1900 tuberculosis (TB) was killing two hundred out of every one hundred thousand Americans. By 1940, just before antibiotics began to be used for treatment, that number had declined to sixty people per one hundred thousand. This decrease was possibly the result of improved sanitation in cities and towns. Because most deaths from TB occurred in urban areas, early treatment consisted of clean, fresh country air. Health spas or sanitoriums that promoted fresh air and quality food were built throughout the European countryside and soon caught on in the United States. Their effect was to act as a quarantine to prevent the spread of tuberculosis. Patients were actually cured or saw their condition improve at the sanitoriums.[12] What does this teach us? Rest, stress reduction, and proper nutrition can boost the immune system and contribute to good health.

Not until TB rates had dropped drastically were antibiotics developed for the treatment of the disease. Even though it was thought that TB would be eliminated, the incidence of tuberculosis has increased 12 percent between 1989 and 1999, possibly due to the emergence of antibiotic-resistant strains of *Mycobacterium tuberculosis*. Because the tuberculosis organism has developed resistance to many antibiotics, patients are often treated with several antibiotics simultaneously.

Another reason the rates of TB have increased is that it is often seen as an opportunistic infection. This means it primarily strikes those who have weakened immune systems and are more vulnerable to disease, such as patients with AIDS, those taking cancer chemotherapy, and those living in crowded conditions. When both tuberculosis and AIDS occur in the same patient, they can aggravate each other, accelerating and worsening both diseases.[13, 14]

Tuberculosis has killed more people than any other pathogen in history and is still killing at an alarming rate, not only in developing countries, but in industrialized nations like the United States as well.

POLIOMYELITIS

Usually referred to as polio or infantile paralysis, this disease was feared by most Americans between 1915 and 1955, when it reached epidemic proportions. This disease of the central nervous system can sometimes cause permanent paralysis in its victims. The virus is found in water supplies and finds its human host through activities such as drinking, bathing, irrigation, and swimming. This is one disease that ironically worsened to epidemic proportions due to improved sanitation and hygiene. Very few infected people actually contract the disease. In fact, for every one thousand infected individuals, only one to three actually show clinical symptoms; the rest develop a natural immunity to the disease. With improvements in sanitation and cleaner water supplies, the reservoir for disease contact became limited. The result of this, however, was that infants and children were coming in contact with the virus less frequently, so that the age at which a person became infected gradually began to increase from infancy to adulthood. The older the victim is, the more chance he or she will become clinically ill from the disease and be paralyzed, rather than develop an immunity to the disease.[15]

The Salk and Sabin vaccines against polio, developed in 1955 and 1960, respectively, brought back the immunization of infants. The United States has not seen a polio case since 1994 and is declared to be polio-free. This should soon be reflected in a change in infant immunization requirements.[16]

INFLUENZA

Although it is a common and mild disease in most people, influenza can worsen to pneumonia, with fatal consequences. It is a highly communicable disease, with school-aged children responsible for the majority of transmission. Epidemics in the United States usually appear during the winter months. Some types of influenza virus find a reservoir in animals, where they can wait it out until finding a human host. (This is why it is also referred to as the swine flu.) Pandemics of the disease tend to be cyclical, occurring every ten to forty years, allowing time for new subtypes to appear. Influenza was at its worst in 1918, when the Spanish flu killed an estimated twenty-one million people worldwide. In 1957, 1968, and 1977 flu pandemics again were seen.[17]

Treating and preventing influenza is arduous because of the virus's characteristic of constantly changing or mutating so that each year it behaves as if it is a totally different virus. This ability works to the virus's advantage, allowing it to continue to find hosts in which to reproduce. Although each time we get the flu we develop immunity to that strain of the virus and cannot become reinfected with that particular virus, the same virus rarely strikes twice and there is no cross-immunity to other influenza viruses. Because of this, the vaccine for influenza is a different one each year, and is based on suggestions from the World Health Organization and the U.S. Public Health Service. It is essentially a gamble as to whether the viruses selected are the ones that will cause influenza that season. This makes the vaccines effective for only one flu season, requiring revaccination annually. These vaccines are no more than 70 percent effective and have some side effects. These include severe allergic reactions and occasionally a neurological disease called Guillain-Barré syndrome.[18] The vaccine is also less effective in people over the age of sixty. In the United States this vaccine has been recommended for all people over sixty-five years of age, those with chronic heart or lung disease, residents of nursing homes, and those in a position to transfer the disease to these high-risk groups, such as medical personnel.

Although older antiviral drugs seemed to have little effect against the influenza virus, in 1999 two new drugs were introduced; oseltamivir (Tamiflu) and zanamivir (Relenza). They belong to a class of drugs called neuraminidase inhibitors. Relatively recent studies have shown that these drugs are effective in treating a number of influenza types but can cause side effects such as nausea, vomiting, bronchitis, and sleep disturbance—the very symptoms of a flu itself.[19] Long-term studies have not yet been conducted to determine side effects that may show up years from now. Because influenza costs us around $12 billion annually[20] from time taken off from work, schools, and day care facilities, drug companies are very interested in developing drugs to combat the disease.

NEW DISEASES

Although Americans' biggest fear at one time might have been Soviet attacks, the greatest worry now apparently is new infectious diseases. We seem to be reading much news of diseases that appear to arise out of nowhere, such as Ebola virus and *Escherichia coli* 0157:H7, both of which progress rapidly to death.[21] Often these diseases are ones that have found a home in an animal and suddenly infect human beings. Because these pathogens have had no time to evolve with humans, they are at first deadly. With time, these pathogens may attenuate and become less deadly to their hosts. It is common for pathogens to lessen in severity with time, as is thought to have happened in the case of the common cold virus. As mentioned earlier, it is in the best interest of the virus to live together with the host rather than to kill it.

LYME DISEASE

Named after a town in Connecticut where the initial cases of the disease were diagnosed, Lyme disease is a consequence of urban sprawl putting more and more suburbanites in contact with ticks. It is caused by a type of bacterium called a spirochete, specifically *Bor-*

relia burgdorferi, which infects deer ticks. A tick bite transmits the bacteria to humans and the result is Lyme disease. This is a chronic disease that can take years to fully manifest itself and has a multitude of symptoms that include neurological problems, cardiac problems, and arthritis. The disease actually evolves in three stages. The first is a simple skin lesion that appears from three days to four weeks after the tick bite. This is a flat, red lesion that slowly grows in size. Flulike symptoms, such as headache, fever, and chills, often accompany the lesion. Weeks to months later, the spirochete infects the blood or lymph fluid, causing more diverse symptoms. These can include additional skin lesions, joint and muscle pain, fatigue, and such neurological symptoms as paralysis in the face. Rarely, cardiac disease and meningitis are present. The third phase does not begin until months or even years after infection. This phase includes more severe skin, joint, and nervous system problems, which become chronic. Nervous system problems comprise memory loss, mood changes, and sleep disturbances. The arthritis can be debilitating.[22]

The typical progression of Lyme disease is not seen in many patients. Symptoms vary widely, but the condition is most commonly mistaken for the flu. In the eastern United States, where the disease is most prevalent, Lyme disease is usually overdiagnosed and treated with antibiotics as a prophylactic approach. A vaccine against Lyme disease was approved in 1998, but with guarded enthusiasm. Lyme disease is noncontagious and nonfatal, but can cause serious organ damage if it is not treated. Lyme disease is best prevented by avoiding contact with ticks. If you frequent the woods, wear protective clothing and check for ticks, both on yourself and on your pets. Lyme disease is not the only disease acquired from ticks; another such tick-borne bacterial disease is human granulocytic ehrlichiosis (also known as erlichia). The symptoms are somewhat similar to those of Lyme disease, but ehrlichia can be fatal.[23]

FLESH-EATING STREP

Since the death in 1990 of Jim Henson, creator of the Muppets, from necrotizing fasciitis, this disease has been sensationalized and referred to as flesh-eating strep. It was first identified in 1924 and was well known during World War II, although it seemed to disappear until the mid-1980s. Necrotizing fasciitis is caused by a more powerful variant of the same type of group A strep that causes strep throat, skin rashes, scarlet fever, and rheumatic fever. This invasive type of group A strep grows quickly under the skin and produces potent toxins that destroy the underlying layer of skin. It can be contracted after abdominal surgery or a minor trauma from an asymptomatic carrier of the bacteria, sometimes producing flulike symptoms initially. With this type of infection, time is of the essence in terms of treatment, and quick-acting antibiotics are necessary to save the patient's life. Sometimes just a few hours' delay can be too long.[24, 25]

LEGIONNAIRES' DISEASE

Named after the American Legion convention held in 1976 in Pennsylvania, which celebrated the bicentennial of the signing of the Declaration of Independence, Legionnaires' disease killed thirty-four people who stayed at the Bellevue-Stratford Hotel in Philadelphia. Detective work discovered that the causative organism, *Legionella pneumophila*, was also the culprit in several previously unidentified deaths. This disease may have existed for years, but had been categorized as an unknown pneumonia. The bacterium tends to live in moist places, including showerheads, hot tubs, steam rooms, fountains, and even grocery store vegetable misters, as well as in ponds and creeks. At the Bellevue-Stratford Hotel, it was in the air-conditioning system—from there it could spread throughout the building.

Patients usually contract the disease by inhaling the organism and develop flulike symptoms, chest and abdominal pains, fever and chills, dry cough, pneumonia, and mental confusion. Death can occur after several weeks. To minimize the presence of the organism, all water-holding devices need to be cleaned thoroughly. The disease is not spread from person to person.[26, 27]

EBOLA

Both the Ebola and Marburg viruses are also referred to as the African hemorrhagic fevers and can cause a gruesome death from bleeding, claiming up to 90 percent of their victims. The first signs are headache, fever, and muscle pain. The most serious Ebola outbreaks occurred in Zaire in 1976 and 1995; three other outbreaks occurred since then in Gabon. Another possible outbreak occurred in 1999 in the Congo. Each of these outbreaks was a slightly different subtype of Ebola. The natural host for Ebola is thought to be monkeys, as many cases have been linked to people who ate or handled monkeys that were infected with the disease. Although it was once thought to be the next great threat to humanity, Ebola no longer appears to have the capability to spread worldwide as an epidemic. The virus causes such an acute infection that it kills its victim very rapidly, sometimes within a week. By doing so, the virus actually harms its own long-term survival by destroying the host it needs to live off. This prevents it from spreading rapidly within a population. The Marburg virus, which infected thirty-one people and killed seven in Germany in 1967, appears to be related to Ebola and was traced to a shipment of monkeys infected with the virus that arrived from Uganda.[28, 29]

LASSA FEVER

Another virus that has been responsible for outbreaks of hemorrhagic disease in western Africa over the last twenty-five years is the Lassa virus. The normal host is a rat, and it is thought that the disease is spread to humans by rat urine coming in contact with open skin. Victims of the disease initially display flulike symptoms and then deteriorate rapidly. Widespread cellular damage occurs, and death due to cardiac failure comes quickly. The disease is not highly contagious among humans, making it less of a threat than are some of the other viruses. In 1989, two outbreaks of Lassa fever occurred in hospitals in Nigeria. These cases were caused by unskilled hospital workers who reused syringes and didn't follow proper sterilization procedures.[30, 31]

HANTAVIRUS

Cases of hantavirus have been found in rural areas of the southwestern United States since 1993, but the name originated from the Han River in South Korea. While fighting in the Korean War, U.S. soldiers came down with the disease caused by this virus. Although it is thought that the virus is transmitted to humans by the deer mouse, there are some cases that have not been traced to the mouse. Like many other viruses, the hantavirus begins with flulike symptoms. With this disease, however, the lungs quickly fill with fluid and death follows rapidly, within days.[32]

ACQUIRED IMMUNODEFICIENCY SYNDROME (AIDS)

AIDS was first recognized in 1980 with the rise in cases of *Pneumocystitis carinii* pneumonia (PCP) and Kaposi's sarcoma, both of which were previously quite rare. These diseases primarily affect those with weakened immune systems or immunodeficiencies; for this reason, the condition that gave rise to these manifestations was called acquired immunodeficiency syndrome, or AIDS. This disease is characterized by a weakened immune system, making the body more prone to a variety of otherwise harmless diseases. The number of AIDS cases escalated from 1980 until 1995, at which time AIDS-related illnesses and deaths began to decline, according to the HIV/AIDS Surveillance Report, published by the Centers for Disease Control, suggesting that the epidemic may be in a waning phase.[33]

It took just four years for scientists to isolate a virus from AIDS patients. Credit for the discovery of this retrovirus is given to Robert Gallo of the United States, who called the virus HIV (human immunodeficiency virus). However, the same virus was simultaneously described by Luc Montagnier, of France, and called HTLV (human T-cell leukemia virus). The prevailing theory in the AIDS research community is that the condition is caused by an infection by HIV. However, after fifteen years of research and $14 billion spent, this theory remains unproved and though it may be waning, AIDS is still at epidemic proportions.[34]

HIV is known to infect certain lymphocytes known as helper T cells, or T4 cells, to be more precise. It is thought that this may be what is responsible for weakening the immune system, making the body more prone to infections. Patients then experience weight loss and weakness. It can take seven to ten years from the time of HIV infection until the patient actually has a full-blown case of AIDS. This is one reason that some scientists question the HIV/AIDS theory.

Peter Duesberg, a professor of molecular biology at the University of California at Berkeley, is the main force behind questioning the cause of AIDS. Since 1987, Duesberg has argued that HIV-type 1 does not fulfill Koch's requirements to determine whether a given microbe causes a specific disease. The inconsistencies in the AIDS theory include the fact that there are at least 4,600 cases of people who have died of AIDS but were found not to be infected with HIV. Second, AIDS cannot be duplicated in any experimental animal model. When HIV is injected into chimpanzees, the animals develop antibodies to HIV but never show signs of AIDS. These characteristics could be explained by the fact that HIV is an atypical virus and does not follow the rules previously described for infectious agents. Alternatively, it could mean that HIV infection is not the cause of AIDS but rather one of the symptoms of the disease. Duesberg suggests that the source of AIDS lies in the lifestyle that accompanies long-term consumption of recreational drugs, such as heroin, cocaine, and nitrite inhalants. Ninety-five percent of AIDS victims in the United States engage in some type of high-risk behavior. These habits also lead to lack of sleep and malnutrition. Combined, they destroy the immune system. Although Duesberg does not claim to have all the answers, he is suggesting that research look at alternatives to the HIV theory.[35]

At present AIDS is diagnosed by the presence of the HIV antibody and a low T-lymphocyte count, which eliminates the possibility of diagnosing the disease in people not infected with HIV—further contributing to the misunderstanding of AIDS. Despite high hopes, research has yet to provide a cure or a vaccine for AIDS.[36]

NORMAL FLORA

The body is host to a multitude of bacteria living in microenvironments of the body. These bacteria live harmoniously with us without causing harm or influencing anatomy, physiology, and susceptibility to pathogenic organisms. These organisms are referred to as normal flora. *Flora* denotes the plants of a specific area, but in this case the word pertains to bacteria rather than plants. In fact, there are probably more bacteria associated with the body than there are cells of the body itself. These bacteria help digest food in the intestines and even produce additional nutrients that are used by the host. Most important, they compete with pathogenic organisms for space, keeping their numbers low. At times, however, normal bacteria can be harmful— for example, by causing dental caries and abscesses.

The human body is first introduced to its normal flora during birth, and bacterial growth continues in an orderly sequence until most of the body is populated with normal flora. Normal flora is acquired from the mother and other people with whom the infant comes in contact. The greatest number of bacteria are found in the large intestines, followed by the mouth. Which bacteria inhabit a specific area of the body is determined by the particularities of the environment—the pH, the temperature, and the amount of oxygen, moisture, and other nutrients. Gram-positive organisms are dominant in the gastrointestinal tracts of breast-fed babies. This balance changes to gram-negative organisms when a baby is bottle-fed.

SKIN

Bacteria live in the outer layers of the epidermis. The types vary somewhat, depending on such factors as moisture, and air, but most of the skin contains *Staphylococcus epidermidis. Staphylococcus aureus* resides on moist areas of the skin, such as the nose and perineum, and can be a common cause of skin diseases. The next most common skin bacteria, primarily on the mucous membranes, are the corynebacteria, or diphtheroids. Although most of them are harmless, the organism that causes diphtheria is a member of this family. Besides these organisms, there are yeasts and even microscopic mites that inhabit the skin and the hair follicles. Fungal spores also tend to take root under fingernails and toenails, where they can then cause infection. The streptococci rarely are found on the skin, except in cases where they are causing disease. Many strep species, however, are found in the mouth, and these can spread to the skin.[37]

UPPER RESPIRATORY TRACT AND MOUTH

Remember that the role of the nose is to act as a filter, removing any unwanted particles from the air before they reach the lungs. Thus, the nose is a dirt trap containing innumerable bacteria, mostly corynebacteria and staphylococci. Many people carry pathogenic strep and staph bacteria in their noses, spreading these bacteria to others through the air.

The types of organisms in the mouth change throughout life. Although there are more than four hundred species of bacteria living in the mouth, most of the surfaces of the mouth are covered with streptococcal species. These bacteria, as well as several anaerobic (not requiring oxygen) bacteria, establish themselves in the mouth early in life. When the teeth come in, the spirochetes *Prevotella* and *Fusobacterium* become entrenched. Later in life, some of these bacteria are the cause of dental disease, including cavities (also known as caries), gingivitis, and periodontal disease.

Organisms in the upper windpipe are usually similar to those found in the mouth. High doses of penicillin are known to change the balance here, eradicating the gram-positive organisms, allowing gram-negative organisms to grow. These gram-negative organisms include *E. coli* and *Pseudomonas,* which are more likely to cause disease. The lower respiratory tract and lungs are normally free of bacteria, except in the case of infection. Aspirating or inhaling bacteria from the mouth can be a cause of pneumonia or lung abscesses.[28]

DIGESTIVE TRACT

The digestive tract is germ-free at birth, but soon becomes home to a number of bacteria. Because of its hostile environment, however, the stomach usually contains no or few bacteria. Bacteria that are swallowed with food are typically killed by stomach acids and enzymes. The exception is *Helicobacter pylori,* which infects the stomach lining and can cause gastritis and ulcers. Food is rapidly pushed forward through the small intestine, minimizing the number of bacteria there.

When you get as far as the large intestine, however, changes in pH favor more bacteria. In fact, more bacteria live in the large intestine than anywhere else in the human body. The most plentiful, and thankfully the most beneficial, bacteria in the intestines are the gram-positive *Bifidobacteria* and *Lactobacilli* organisms. They are able to produce such acids as acetic acid, butyric acid, and lactic acid. These

by-products enhance health in a number of ways including preventing cancer, stimulating immunity, and inhibiting the growth of
pathogenic bacteria in the intestines.[39] Babies that are bottle-fed,
however, have fewer of these beneficial bacteria.

The types of bacteria change as you go farther into the intestines. In a normal adult there are more than one hundred different
types of bacteria in the intestines, among them *Bacteroides, Fusobacterium, Clostridia,* and *E. coli.* Together the organisms of the intestines
provide the body with vitamin K, absorb nutrients from the intestines, and compete with microbial pathogens in the intestines. When
the balance of beneficial organisms in the intestinal tract is altered—
for example, by ingestion of antimicrobial drugs—abscesses and
peritonitis, among others diseases, can occur. Organisms such as
Clostridium difficile become dominant. This shift in the balance of
power can also lead to nutrient deficiencies by limiting vitamin B_{12}
uptake. *Candida* organisms are also normal residents there; they cause
problems only when their growth is out of balance. This can happen
if the number of gram-positive bacteria declines for some reason,
allowing *Candida* organisms to take hold.[40]

UROGENITAL TRACT

The outer genital area, or vulva, harbors bacteria similar to those
found on the skin. Often, owing to the presence of moisture, this
area also is home to gram-negative bacteria. Several factors regulate
the type of bacteria common to the vagina: pH, age, and hormone
levels. Near puberty, the pH of the vagina drops, becoming acidic.
At this time, *Lactobacillus acidophilus,* corynebacteria, pepto-
streptococci, staphylococci, streptococci, and *Bacteroides* species are
common. At menopause, the pH of the vagina increases, becoming
alkaline. It is easier for yeasts to dominate, which can cause vaginitis. Bacteria are usually not found in the bladder and urethra because the flow of urine constantly washes out any bacteria that find
their way up this passage. At the outer opening of the urethra, however, *S. epidermidis,* enterococci, and diphtheroids are common;
E. coli, Proteus, and *Neisseria* organisms can also be found there. All
of these bacteria coexist in the body to provide optimum health.[41]

If this delicate balance is altered by damage to the skin, antibiotics that kill off some of the normal flora, or the introduction of a large amount of pathogenic bacteria, the result can be infection. This may also happen with a weakened immune system or the buildup of damaged tissue caused by overall poor health, which serves as a breeding ground for pathogens.

TABLE 1. COMMON DISEASE-CAUSING BACTERIA

Gram-positive bacteria	Disease
Bacillus anthracis	Anthrax
Clostridium, spp.	Wound infections (gangrene), tetanus, botulism
Corynebacterium diphtheriae	Diphtheria
Enterococcus	Wound infections, urinary tract infections, endocarditis
Staphylococcus aureus	Skin infections, such as folliculitis; wound infections; rarely, osteomyelitis; blood infections; and toxic shock syndrome. *S. aureus* is a common hospital-acquired infection, especially when intravenous devices are used.
Staphylococcus spp., e.g., *S. epidermis*	Wound infections and hospital-acquired infections from surgery and the use of internal prostheses, such as cardiac valves and dialysis catheters
Streptococcus— group A beta-hemolytic	Strep throat; impetigo; rarely, necrotizing fasciitis
Streptococcus—non-group A	Sore throat, impetigo
Streptococcus pneumoniae	Pneumonia, meningitis

Gram-negative bacteria	Disease
Actinomyces israelii	Abscesses in the mouth, gastrointestinal tract, or lungs
Bartonella (Rochalimaea) henselae	Cat-scratch disease
Bordetella pertussis	Whooping cough
Brucella spp.	Brucellosis (contracted from animals)
Campylobacter spp.	Systemic infections, blood infections, and meningitis associated with drinking raw, contaminated milk
Chlamydiae spp.	Genital and urinary tract infections. One species causes psittacosis, a lung infection contracted from birds.
Escherichia coli (E. coli)	Gastroenteritis. Some strains are more toxic than others. The strain 0157:H7, from undercooked hamburger and unpasteurized juice, has caused death in young children.
Francisella (Pasteurella) tularensis	Tularemia (contracted from wild rodents)
Haemophilus influenzae	Sinusitis, ear infections, bronchitis, pneumonia, arthritis, meningitis
Legionella pneumophila	Legionnaires' disease
Mycobacterium leprae	Leprosy
Mycobacterium tuberculosis	Tuberculosis
Neisseria gonorrhoeae	Gonococcal infection (venereal disease)

Gram-negative bacteria	Disease
Neisseria meningitidis	Meningitis
Nocardia spp.	Nocardiosis (lung infection)
Prevotella (Bacteroides) melaninogenica, Bacteroides fragilis	Periodontal infection, pneumonia, intra-abdominal infections, pelvic infections
Salmonella enterica	Salmonellosis (gastroenteritis), typhoid fever, blood infections
Shigella sonnei, S.flexneri, S.dysenteriae	Shigellosis (dysentery)
Vibrio cholerae	Cholera. Other species of *Vibrio* cause food poisoning from contaminated fish.
Yersinea pestis	Plague (contracted from wild rodents)

2 IMMUNOLOGY

HOW DOES THE BODY
PROTECT ITSELF FROM DISEASE?

Why do we get infections? There are two theories. The germ theory developed by Pasteur states that bacteria cause infection. The second theory, that of Metchnikoff, holds that infections are the result of a weak host. In truth, both of these factors probably work together to cause infection. Microorganisms are part of the human body, living on our skin and in our intestines and mouth. Very rarely do they cause disease. There are many factors that make one person less susceptible to infectious disease than others, including elements that we can control, such as diet, nutrition, lifestyle, stress, and environment, as well as things that we cannot control, like heredity. When infection strikes, the body has many ways in which to react. In fact, there are three levels of protection the body uses. These are physical barriers formed by the skin, lungs, digestive tract, and urinary tract; inflammation; and immunity.[1]

Physical Barriers

Skin

Skin wraps around the entire body, preventing infectious agents from entering. It is also home to some cells of the immune system. If the skin does not remain intact, however, such as when we suffer cuts, bacteria can enter the body at that place and increase the chance of infection.

The skin is made up of two main layers: The epidermis is the outermost layer and the dermis is the inner layer. A third layer, the subcutaneous layer, lies beneath the dermis. The epidermal layer consists of flat, thin epithelial cells. They make a large protein called keratin, which gives the skin strength, makes it waterproof, and protects it from many chemicals. The cells in the epidermis are constantly regenerating themselves. In fact, every thirty days or so the skin is completely replaced owing to the growth of new cells. As new cells divide, they push the older ones upward or away from the body. Even after these outer cells die, they are still important because their high level of keratin provides much protection to the epidermis. Eventually, these cells slough off as new ones continue to grow. This shedding of cells also removes microorganisms on the surface of the skin.

The outer layer of skin is slightly acidic, which prevents the growth of bacteria on the skin. Washing with alkaline soaps removes this protective acid layer. After washing your face, it is a good idea to use a low-pH toner, which will restore the acid layer. (*See* chapter 9 for a recipe for herbal vinegar toner.) The skin also secretes certain substances that keep bacteria at bay.

The dermis, located under the epidermis, is the thickest layer of skin. The dermis is connective tissue, made up of such proteins as collagen and elastin. These proteins give the skin flexibility and the ability to stretch, as during pregnancy or in the case of obesity or water retention. The thickness of the dermis varies; it is thickest on the palms and soles of the feet and very thin on the eyelids and scrotum. The dermis is rich with blood vessels, nerves, sweat glands, oil glands, and hair follicles. Underneath is the subcutaneous layer, made up of fat, which insulates, protects, and connects the skin to the muscles.

Imagine running and falling down on a knee. Part of the skin is scraped away. This type of a wound, or abrasion, affects just the upper layer of skin—the epidermis. Healing begins immediately. First, basal cells at the lower portion of the epidermis become larger and begin to glide across any area where the dermis is exposed. Covering the dermis provides immediate protection to the body. At the same time, proteins are released at the wound site, and this causes the cells to begin dividing so that they can fill in the gap left by cells that were removed from the epidermis. Remember, there are no blood vessels in the epidermis, so there is no bleeding from a minor abrasion and healing is usually complete after two days. If healing does not take place quickly, the normal bacteria found on the skin can start to cause an infection at the site. (*See* chapter 9 for a recipe for a balm to help promote this healing and prevent infection.)

If a wound goes deeper into the skin, to the dermal layer, healing is more complicated. The first response will be inflammation, which causes redness, pain, swelling, and heat in the skin. Although your first thought might be to stop the inflammation, keep in mind that the role of inflammation is to prevent bacteria from growing at the site and to remove any dead and damaged tissue.

Blood clotting also begins immediately. Because the dermal layer is rich with blood vessels, varying degrees of bleeding will take place with a deep cut. A scab then forms from the dried blood, filling in the area of skin that is open. Don't pick off this scab, or you will expose the wound again. Epithelial cells of the skin move under the scab and begin dividing to close the opening. More cells from the dermis, called fibroblasts, grow and form scar tissue. The scar tissue will be more dense and contain fewer blood vessels and hair and sensory nerves. After enough epithelial cells have grown to close the wound, the scab is pushed off and healing is complete.

LUNGS

Although the main job of the lungs, or respiratory tract, is to exchange oxygen for carbon dioxide, they also play an important role in keeping out infectious agents. As air first enters the nose, it is warmed, moistened, and filtered. Coarse hairs in the nose bar the entrance of large dust particles that may contain infectious agents, while mucus moistens the air and also traps dust particles. The air tubes that extend from the back of the mouth into the lungs are called the trachea and the bronchial tubes. The cells that line these tubes have tiny hairs, or cilia, on their surfaces that spread out to catch small particles that are able to make their way past the nose. These tiny cilia move back and forth, pushing bacteria and other particles up and out of the lungs. The sticky mucus in this area also helps trap bacteria to keep it out of the lungs. Cigarette smoke can paralyze the cilia, preventing them from doing their job. This is one of the reasons that smokers are much more prone to respiratory diseases.

As the tubes into the lungs become smaller and cilia are no longer present, specialized white blood cells called macrophages can remove inhaled particles that find their way lower into the lungs. Mucus that lines the bronchial tubes also helps trap infectious particles, preventing them from interacting with the cells of the body. Coughing removes particles that have made it past this level of protection to the lungs.

DIGESTIVE TRACT

Saliva washes the mouth and teeth, keeping them clean. It dilutes the microbes there but also has the ability to kill or damage bacteria. As food passes into the stomach, it enters a very acidic liquid, which helps turn food into liquid but also works to destroy bacteria, keeping them from growing. If that isn't enough, enzymes used for digesting food also inhibit the growth of microbes.

Finally, when food passes into the intestines, protective mechanisms there help prevent infection. As nutrients from the food are absorbed, they first enter the lymphatic system rather than traveling directly into the blood. The lymphatic system then has the opportunity to filter out microbes before they penetrate the blood. Mucus in the intestines also helps trap any microbes that have made it that far. Even with all this protection, if large numbers of bacteria enter the body through contaminated food, infection can take root.

URINARY TRACT

Protection provided by the urinary tract is similar to the previous examples. The tissue that lines the urinary tract is a physical barrier to microbes. As urine passes through the urethra to the outside of the body, it washes away microbes that may have entered the urethra from the skin. The acid pH of the urine also provides protection from infection by inhibiting bacterial growth.

INFLAMMATION

As good as they are, it is still possible for an invading microbe to make it through the physical barriers provided by the skin and by other tissue that lines the passages into the body. When this happens, the second level of protection comes into play. Inflammation, as we already discussed, is what occurs when skin is scraped. It involves a large number of chemicals that cause redness, pain, swelling, and heat. Remember, inflammation is a positive response, but for healing to continue, inflammation must eventually stop. If it persists longer than necessary, it will block the healing process.

Inflammation works in the following way. When you cut your finger, the damaged skin starts making several chemicals that travel into the blood, alerting the body to possible danger. The body has a number of responses. The damaged area becomes hot, which increases metabolism to speed healing. Swelling occurs, bringing more nutrients to the area to promote healing. Specialized white blood cells—macrophages—invade the area and remove microbes and damaged tissue. Blood clotting takes place. All of these actions decrease the chances of an infectious agent taking hold.

Some other chemicals that are involved in this second line of defense are described in table 2. All of these mechanisms work together to prevent pathogenic bacteria from reproducing enough to gain a foothold and cause disease. Inflammation is not just a localized response. It can affect the entire body when responding to a larger-scale infection. In this case, the heat takes the form of fever.

TABLE 2. CHEMICALS INVOLVED IN INFLAMMATION[2]

Chemical	Action
Complement	Attaches to the bacteria cell membrane, causing rupture
Histamine	Causes small blood vessels or capillaries to swell with blood
Interferons	Stop the spread of a virus from one cell to another
Prostaglandins	Cause the sensation of pain
Pyrogens	Act on the brain to bring about a fever

THE IMMUNE SYSTEM

The body has another card to play when inflammation is not sufficient to counter infection. When microbes are able to penetrate the first and second levels of defense and successfully produce infection, the body's immune system is activated. This is a very specialized response that involves a complex system of cells and chemicals directed at a specific foreign antigen. This process probably evolved in human beings when infectious diseases first began to appear. Without the immune system, we would not survive. Keeping it functioning at optimum efficiency is essential to both ward off infections and control cancer.

The immune system basically is made up of white blood cells, also called leukocytes. They are produced in the bone marrow and circulate throughout the blood vessels as well as the lymph system. The lymph system includes lymph vessels as well as such organs as the spleen, appendix, thymus, tonsils, and many small lymph nodes. The different types of white blood cells are listed in table 3.

TABLE 3. TYPES OF WHITE BLOOD CELLS

White blood cell type	Concentration in blood (number of cells/mm3)	Function
Basophils	20–50	Make and release histamine
Eosinophils	100–400	Primarily involved in parasitic infection as well as allergies
Lymphocytes	1,500–3,000	Varied roles, including making antibodies and directly attacking microbes; include T cells and B cells
Macrophages	N.A.	Specialized monocytes found in tissues rather than in the blood
Monocytes	100–700	Digest debris, bacteria, and damaged cells found in the blood
Neutrophils	3,000–7,000	Phagocytize or "eat" bacteria

The role of the immune system is to determine what belongs to the body and what doesn't. When it perceives something as being "not self," it acts by destroying and removing it. This is quite a job! Besides identifying and removing microbes, the immune system must identify and remove cells of its own body that have transformed to become cancerous. It also recognizes organ transplants, which is why patients who have received transplants must take potent drugs to suppress the immune system and prevent rejection of the transplant. This reaction, of course, makes them much more prone to both infection and cancer. Cells of the immune system recognize foreign elements in the body by a code on the cell surface that they detect as not part of the body, or "not self." This code takes the form of an antigen, which can be proteins or large polysaccharides present on the surface of a foreign cell or virus.

Understanding the immune system has proved to be a major medical advance of the twentieth century. As early as the late 1800s, the Russian scientist Élie Metchnikoff used a microscope to observe the white blood cells from infected animals in the process of eating, or phagocytizing, disease substances. From this observation he developed the theory of cellular immunity, which holds that white blood cells are responsible for developing immunity, or exemption from a certain disease.[3] At the same time, scientists from Germany were proposing a chemical theory for immunity. Three German scientists led the way in developing this theory: Robert Koch, Emil Adolf von Behring, and Paul Ehrlich. They argued that blood serum was responsible for immunity—this became known as the humoral theory of immunity.

We now know that both theories are correct, existing side by side and supporting each other. The cellular immune system comprises the actions of the immune cells themselves in destroying foreign cells, and the humoral immune system refers to the soluble chemicals produced by these cells that destroy alien cells. Lymphocytes, in fact, are involved in both types of immune systems, but in differing ways. These parallel systems are summarized in table 4. Lymphocytes begin to reproduce and increase in numbers when they detect the presence of a foreign antigen. Two different types of lymphocytes respond, each to a slightly different stimulus. B lymphocytes respond to microorganisms; T lymphocytes respond to the body's own cells that have changed. Such change could be due to mutations that might lead to cancer or to invasion by a virus. The T lymphocytes can also respond to larger microorganisms, such as fungi and parasites. It is the action of the B lymphocytes, or the B-cell response, that falls into the category of humoral immunity, whereas the action of T lymphocytes, or the T-cell response, is called cell-mediated immunity.[4]

CELL-MEDIATED IMMUNITY

Cell-mediated immunity is driven by the T cells' direct interaction with a foreign cell, rather than through the production of antibodies. They are termed "T" cells because they mature in the thymus gland. When a T cell senses a foreign antigen on the surface of a cell, it destroys that cell. That foreign cell can be one of the body's own cells that has mutated as the result of cancer or viral infection, a fungus, a bacterium, or a parasite. There are subcategories of T cells, which include helper T cells and killer T cells. Once the helper T cell identifies a foreign cell in the body, it goes to the spleen and lymph nodes looking for other cells that can help, either T or B cells. The HIV virus associated with AIDS infects these helper T cells, also called T4 cells. When these cells are destroyed, the victim becomes immunocompromised and is then much more prone to a variety of infections.

Once a killer T cell is activated by the helper T cell, it is ready to kill abnormal cells (such as viral-infected and cancerous cells). Finally, when the infection has been wiped out and is no longer a threat to the body, a third type of T cell, the suppressor T cell, helps the immune system shut down. This step is vital in allowing the body to begin to repair tissue damage that may have been caused by the infection.

HUMORAL IMMUNITY

B cells, so called because they develop in the bursa of Fabricius in birds, or in the bone marrow of human beings, produce proteins called antibodies. Once activated by the helper T cells, the B cells look for foreign cells by identifying foreign antigens on a cell surface. In a way, these surface antigens are like addresses that indicate whether the cell belongs in the body. When a foreign antigen is detected, the B cell can make huge quantities of corresponding antibody.

Antibodies, also called immunoglobulins, are unique proteins made specifically to react with a given antigen. Once made, these antibodies are released from the B cell to circulate in the blood. There they can find and bind with or stick to the corresponding antigen. This action essentially locks up the antigen, preventing it from binding to the body's own cells, where it can cause harm. Eventually this antigen-antibody unit is removed from the bloodstream by a type of white blood cell called the macrophage. These cells all work together in cooperation to keep the body healthy.

It is the humoral immune system that provides the body with long-term resistance or immunity to a disease. Certain white blood cells called memory cells retain the ability to produce antibodies to a given antigen. When the body comes in contact with that foreign antigen, these memory cells are ready to begin making antibodies again, to protect the body from the pathogen. This is the theory behind vaccinations. A foreign antigen is introduced to the body, which then produces antibodies directed against that antigen and stores the information. Antibodies can also be administered directly to a patient to induce passive immunity. These antibodies are formed in another host, purified, and then injected into a patient. This approach is sometimes used when people are exposed to hepatitis.

Both immune systems have the capacity to overreact, causing harm to the body. This is referred to as hypersensitivity, or an allergic reaction. This reaction is the result of the release of histamine and prostaglandins from cells. If the response is immediate, mediated by humoral immunity, it can result in anaphylactic shock and death if not treated. Less serious but nonetheless chronic manifestations include asthma, eczema, destruction of red blood cells, and such autoimmune diseases as arthritis and kidney disease. If the response is delayed, mediated by cellular immunity, the result manifests hours or days later and lasts for several days. This category includes such skin reactions as contact dermatitis caused by poison ivy.

The white blood cells also secrete various chemicals that help in protecting and healing the body. Because of the amount of research done on these chemicals, they are beginning to become common terms to many people. Collectively they are given the name cytokines. Some of these cytokines are reviewed in table 5.

TABLE 4. CELLULAR AND HUMORAL IMMUNITIES

Cellular immunity	Humoral immunity
Mediated by cells	Mediated by antibodies
Involves T cells	Involves B cells
Effective against fungal, viral, and bacterial infections as well as cancer	Effective against toxins, viruses, some microbial infections
Interacts directly with foreign cell	Interacts directly with antigen
Responsible for cell-mediated (delayed) hypersensitivity	Responsible for anaphylactic shock (immediate hypersensitivity)

TABLE 5. CYTOKINES

Specific cytokine	Action
Interferon alpha and beta (IFN-α and IFN-ß)	Inhibit viral replication
Interferon gamma (IFN-γ)	Secreted by activated T cells to activate phagocytes
Interleukin-1 (IL-1)	Secreted by macrophages to attract white blood cells to the site of inflammation; induces fever.
Interleukin-2 (IL-2)	Secreted by T cells to activate other T cells
Transforming growth factor beta (TGF-ß)	Increases inflammation and modulates the development of T and B cells.
Tumor necrosis factor (TNF)	Secreted by T and B cells to attract macrophages to stimulate phagocytosis; has antiviral action and induces fever

KEEPING THE IMMUNE SYSTEM HEALTHY

No one is sure why the immune system works most of the time but at times doesn't work, allowing us to become infected and sick. Sometimes it seems as if we know a lot about the immune system, and sometimes it seems the opposite. Why does the immune system protect us from disease at one time but not always? Why does it overreact, causing allergic responses? Why, sometimes, does it fail to recognize self as self and attack the body's own tissue, causing diseases such as lupus? Keeping the immune system functioning at capacity is important to overall health. We know that alcohol, cigarette smoke, narcotics, and alterations in metabolism that change the pH of the blood have a negative effect on the immune system. Overuse of antibiotics alters the ratio of good to bad bacteria, especially in the gut, which can lead to disease. Improper nutrition weakens the immune system. We ingest many things today that are not nutrients, such as preservatives and pesticides. Each of these affects the immune system. Foreign agents in the environment also have effects. Eating processed foods strips us of micronutrients that support the immune system, including zinc and vitamin C. Many other lifestyle factors cause stress to our bodies, as well, including lack of sleep and exercise, drug use, lack of fresh air, excess artificial light, job changes, and moves. A healthy lifestyle is the key to a healthy immune system.

3 CONTROL
OF INFECTIONS

VACCINATIONS AND IMMUNITY

In the 1790s the English physician Edward Jenner was told by a milk-maid that because she had cowpox, she could not get smallpox. Although this was a well-known phenomenon among milkmaids—and something of a relief to them—physicians had yet to make the connection. Rather than dismiss her statement as being silly, Jenner spent years observing this trend until he was sufficiently convinced that cowpox did provide immunity against smallpox. He then removed pus from a cowpox sore on a dairymaid and scratched it onto the arm of an eight-year-old boy. Jenner waited seven weeks for immunity to develop and then inoculated the boy with smallpox. The boy failed to contract smallpox, even after he was inoculated several times over a number of years. This persuaded many people to become vaccinated against smallpox in a similar manner. In fact, very soon after the initial experiment, vaccination for smallpox became compulsory. In humans, cowpox causes fever, nausea, and sores, but it is not a serious disease. Smallpox vaccinations are no longer given because it was determined in 1978 that smallpox had been eradicated. Because the virus is so stable, however, there exists the possibility of contracting the disease from archaeological artifacts.

The term *vaccination* is from the Latin word for cow, as this first vaccine was derived from cowpox. Vaccinations are a means of providing immunity or resistance to a disease. The word *immunity* originally meant "exempt from" and referred to taxes or military service. As knowledge of infectious disease evolved, however, the word came to be used in reference to those who were protected from foreign substances or diseases. Immunity can be innate or acquired. *Innate* means that resistance has evolved by means of natural selection. For instance, people who live in or are from Africa have developed several forms of resistance to malaria. These are primarily changes in the red blood cells, which make it difficult for a malaria parasite to reproduce there. Sickle cell trait is one example. Although the sickle cell trait saves people from the deadly *Plasmodium* malaria parasite, sickle cell disease itself can be deadly. The difference between sickle cell trait and disease conditions lies in whether a person has inherited one or two genes for that characteristic, or is heterozygous or homozygous for sickle cell.

Acquired immunity generally develops after a person has been exposed to a disease, and it usually results in a lifelong immunity to the disease, preventing the person from again becoming sick from the same microorganism. Developing acquired immunity depends on specialized white blood cells called memory cells—B cells that remain in the body after an infection. They are ready to quickly respond on seeing a virus or antigen for the second time. This response either prevents the disease entirely or causes it to manifest in a milder form. As populations build up these antibodies, what could be a deadly disease lessens to a milder form. Over time within a given community, a compromise is reached whereby the pathogen allows most infected humans to live and, in turn, those infected pass that pathogen along to other people or hosts. In the days of exploration, it was the ability of populations to build up immunities to certain diseases that caused the diseases to become epidemics in other populations. To reach adulthood, explorers naturally had to survive several diseases, which strengthened their immune systems. They were possibly unknowing carriers of these diseases and brought them to conquered populations. Because these populations had never been exposed to these particular diseases, they had not built up any immunity to them and the diseases decimated them.

Vaccinations, also called immunizations, developed as a means of preventing a disease by mimicking this acquired immunity. Introducing the antigen from a disease-causing organism to the body causes a person to form antibodies to protect from the disease.

As early as the eleventh century, Chinese doctors had a crude method of vaccinating against smallpox. They made a powder from the dried scabs of patients with mild cases of smallpox, which was inhaled by healthy patients. Because the dried scabs from smallpox patients contained the smallpox virus, inhaling the powder exposed the healthy people to the virus. Another procedure was to rub scab powder onto a wound inflicted on the skin of the healthy person. The problem with these types of vaccinations is that there is no way to control how serious the disease will become in the healthy patient.

Vaccines are made today by a variety of methods. One is to inject attenuated viruses, or viruses that have become weakened in some way. When a person is injected with a weakened virus, that person may become slightly ill, but not deadly ill. Early vaccines made in this manner include chicken cholera, anthrax, and rabies, all of which were developed by Louis Pasteur. Other methods of vaccine development used a virus after first killing it by heat. Newer methods use a single isolated antigen from the virus.

ARE VACCINES REALLY SAFE AND EFFECTIVE?

In 1999, the American Academy of Pediatrics, the Advisory Committee on Immunization Practices of the Centers for Disease Control and Prevention, and the American Academy of Family Physicians recommended that all children receive the following immunizations:

- Diphtheria, pertussis, and tetanus (usually given together as DPT)
- Haemophilus influenza type b (HIb)
- Hepatitis B

- Measles-mumps-rubella (given together as MMR)
- Polio, recently changed to allow use of the inactivated virus
- Rotavirus
- Varicella (chicken pox)[1]

With this schedule, for a child to be completely vaccinated requires fourteen to nineteen shots by the age of sixteen! While in the past vaccinations have been started at the age of two months, they are now being recommended to begin twelve hours after birth. Despite the highly publicized vaccine campaign in this country, only 40 percent of two-year-olds have all of their recommended shots. Some of this is due to economics, but some of it is due to the ever-increasing concern that parents have regarding the number of vaccines they are being asked to give to their children. No longer are vaccines recommended only to protect against the deadly and crippling diseases such as smallpox and polio, but now vaccines are also administered against relatively mild diseases to prevent economic losses accrued by parents being away from work.

The varicella or chicken pox vaccine, which was introduced in 1995, has several unanswered questions pertaining to it. Chicken pox is a relatively mild childhood disease, and those who contract it as children develop lifelong immunity to it; that is, they become unable to contract the disease again. The vaccine, however, does not provide lifelong immunity, so the possibility of driving the disease into the adult population exists. When contracted as an adult, chicken pox can be a much more serious disease with complications and even deaths. Additionally, the varicella vaccine is a live virus. This means that the risk of contracting disease from the vaccine is greater than if a nonlive virus was used. Because chicken pox is caused by a herpesvirus, this live virus could lie dormant in the body for years, causing shingles later in life.[2] This may be a high price to pay for preventing a relatively benign childhood disease.

At the beginning of 1999, the vaccine series for rotavirus was recommended for infants beginning at two months of age. This virus causes diarrhea in children, which is highly treatable in the United States and other developed countries. In July 1999, however, the

Centers for Disease Control (CDC) recommended that the vaccine be postponed while they examined claims that the vaccine causes a serious type of bowel obstruction. After studying the data, the Advisory Committee on Immunization Practices of the CDC recommended that the vaccine be withdrawn from the market. The Wyeth Lederle Vaccines unit of American Home Products Corporation voluntarily requested that all unused vaccines be returned to the manufacturer.[3]

Another vaccine story that developed recently regards the hepatitis B vaccine. This vaccine is recommended for all newborns. However, it seems to have caused more serious side effects than reported cases of the disease. In 1996 alone, 1,081 adverse events were reported to the Federal Drug Administration following injections given to infants younger than age one. Side effects of the vaccine include chronic fatigue syndrome, seizures, autoimmune diseases such as arthritis and lupus, as well as neurological dysfunctions. Several cases of sudden infant death syndrome (SIDS) are also linked to the hepatitis B vaccine. Forty-eight deaths have been reported as a direct result of this vaccine. Those peoples at risk for hepatitis B include intravenous drug users, those having unprotected sex, and health-care workers—not many newborns fit into these groups. Because a newborn's immune system is delicate and not well developed, the effect of a vaccination on that immune system may be devastating. The reason for giving the vaccination at such an early age is basically an issue of compliance. Physicians have the best access to people while mother and baby are still in the hospital following the birth, making vaccination easier at that time. Most parents, after the ordeal of childbirth, are not ready to question the administration of a vaccine. In July 1999 the U.S. Public Health Service and the American Association of Pediatricians called to roll back the administration of hepatitis B vaccine to six months of age rather than give it to newborns. Some pediatric offices are even recommending that physicians wait until adolescence to administer the hepatitis B vaccine. The U.S. Public Health Service has also called for manufacturers to eliminate mercury from vaccines.[4] Mercury, in the form of thimerosal, is used as a preservative in many vaccines and may be responsible for some side effects.

Control of Infections 41

Despite these blows to the vaccine industry, more vaccines are planned. The FDA just approved a pneumococcal vaccine for prevention of bacterial meningitis and blood-borne infection, or bacteremia. It will probably be proposed that this vaccine be administered at two, four, and six months with a booster at twelve to fifteen months.

Besides these new developments, there remain the concerns regarding vaccinations that have been in use for some time. Among the side effects of vaccination are:

- The DPT shot has caused fever, irritability, encephalopathy, brain damage, and even death in rare cases.
- The oral polio vaccine produces polio in about ten people each year (even in previously vaccinated people). In fact, since 1979 the only U.S. cases of polio have been caused by the vaccine itself.
- In the past, polio vaccines have contained a monkey virus, simian virus–number 40 (SV40), that can cause cancer in humans and sometimes an immunodeficiency virus, simian immunodeficiency virus (SIV), similar to HIV. In fact, it has been theorized that this SIV virus has evolved to become the HIV virus, which is related to AIDS, thus making polio vaccine a potential cause of AIDS.[5]
- The pertussis vaccine causes diabetes in mice. We don't know if it also does so in humans.
- Several vaccines, including those against polio, measles, rubella, HIb, hepatitis B, and tetanus, are associated with neurological disorders, such as Guillain-Barré syndrome.
- The MMR vaccine has caused psychosis, encephalitis, and deafness.
- The measles vaccine may result in Crohn's disease, ulcerative colitis, and inflammatory bowel disease.
- The mumps vaccine has caused meningitis, and rates of asthma and insulin-dependent diabetes in children have increased along with mandatory vaccinations.[6]

We have seen the advent of new and unexplained diseases that affect the nervous system since vaccinations have come into use, as well as dramatic increases in others. Among them are attention deficit disorder, autism, criminal behavior among children, and asthma. To establish a definite relationship between neurological and immunological damage and vaccinations would be impossible. Likewise, to prove that there is no relationship is also impossible. Much of the damage caused by vaccines occurs as delayed reactions. These are not officially accounted for as side effects by physicians and vaccine manufacturers; side effects are considered to be those reactions that take place within forty-eight hours of injection. For this reason, it is difficult to determine the true long-term side effects of vaccines.

OTHER VACCINE BLUNDERS

Many early vaccines, including smallpox and yellow fever, resulted in the spread of hepatitis through the use of dirty needles and human blood present in the vaccine. At that time, the connection between dirty needles and disease had not been made, and sterile procedures were not common. Many deaths were caused by these vaccines between 1938 and 1942. In 1955, two hundred people came down with polio, and eleven died as the result of a vaccine that was not completely inactivated. Earlier, in 1902, an experimental vaccine for plague had been contaminated with tetanus, and in 1906 a vaccine for cholera contained the plague bacteria and killed thirteen prisoners. The first flu vaccine of 1976 killed at least twelve people by causing the rare neurological disorder Guillain-Barré syndrome. Scientists later realized that the strain of influenza they were vaccinating against was not as serious as they had thought it was, making the vaccinations unnecessary.

The most widely used vaccine in the world today is the bacille Calmette-Guerin (BCG) vaccine against tuberculosis. The vaccine is made from bacteria closely related to tuberculosis but found in cows rather than humans. Even though it was developed in 1908, it is still not clear how well the vaccine works, and it has not been recommended in the United States. Those who have received this vaccine test positive on tuberculosis skin tests.

HAVE VACCINATIONS DECREASED
DISEASE RATES?

When you look at the data concerning the number of cases of diseases, you find some interesting facts. Take measles, for instance. The death rate attributed to measles reached a high in the early 1900s and fell dramatically, close to zero by the 1940s. The vaccine was introduced after this decline—in the 1960s—and could not have contributed to the dramatic drop in death due to measles. The same can be said for whooping cough. Death rates from this disease were high before 1920, at which time they began to fall rapidly. The vaccine was initiated after this decline, in the 1940s, thereby having little or no effect on the drop in death rate. The vaccine for polio, however, was introduced just as death rates for polio began to fall, thus making it unclear how much of an effect the vaccine itself had.

There remain many unanswered questions regarding vaccinations. We still have little information on how many vaccinations the immune system can act on effectively, to what degree breast milk might inhibit the immunization response, and, most important, the nature of the long-term effects of vaccines. Some scientists and health practitioners are concerned that the use of immunizations may be contributing to the increase in chronic diseases we have seen lately, including cancer, heart disease, and asthma.

Although many alternative practitioners argue against vaccines, there is controversy even among them. The popular alternative physician Andrew Weil advocates the use of childhood vaccinations, saying that it is only because most of us are unfamiliar with these diseases that we consider forgoing vaccination. Other practitioners advise postponing childhood vaccinations until both the immune system and the nervous system have a chance to develop. Dr. Philip Incao is an anthroposophical physician in Denver. (Anthroposophical medicine integrates allopathic practices with alternative practices, and considers an individual's spiritual aspects along with the physical.) Dr. Incao suggests that childhood diseases are necessary to activate the immune system to fight disease later in life.

A Personal Account

Little Nathan was given a clean bill of health and found to be growing normally when he went to the pediatrician's office for his six-month well-baby checkup. However, when he got home, he began to cry persistently. When his mother called the doctor she was told that this was just a normal reaction to the diphtheria, pertussis, and tetanus (DPT) shot he had just received. His condition worsened to the point of collapse. Nathan's mother called 911, but by the time medical help arrived, the boy was dead. It wasn't until after Nathan's death that his parents began reading up on the side effects of the pertussis (or whooping cough) vaccine, which include high-pitched and persistent screaming, fever, convulsions, and collapse that can lead to brain damage or death.

Although his death was officially attributed to congestive heart failure, Nathan's parents were awarded compensation from the national Vaccine Compensation Program. Nathan's was not the only death. Nine other children were killed, apparently from the same batch of DPT vaccine that Nathan received.

Although the new acellular pertussis vaccine now available has fewer side effects, there are still unanswered questions surrounding its use.[7]

There is not enough room here to give the full arguments for and against vaccinations, but please research and consider both sides before immunizing your children. There are many places to go for more information. The magazine *Mothering* routinely publishes articles updating parents on the vaccination controversy. Other places to find information are the National Vaccine Information Center,

Informed Parents Vaccination Home Page, Natural Immunity Information Network, and the American Association of Pediatrics Committee on Infectious Diseases' Red Book.

Keep in mind that although it is the law in most states that children be vaccinated for admission into school, this law is sometimes flexible. All states permit medical exemptions, most states permit religious exemptions, and fifteen states permit philosophical exemptions. In Colorado, a waiver can be signed by a parent for any reason. Because it is difficult to evaluate the ratio of benefits to risks, it should be a parent's informed choice as to whether and when to vaccinate a child.

Vaccinations carry both risks and benefits, and that risk-to-benefit ratio can be determined only by the patient or the patient's parents. Vaccinations are not 100 percent effective. For instance, the vaccine for whooping cough (pertussis) ranges from 63 percent to 94 percent effective. There have been many instances of vaccinated people becoming infected. The Association of American Physicians and Surgeons has called for an end to the government's mandatory vaccination program.[8] With the revenues from sales of vaccines having increased 300 percent since 1986,[9] one wonders what the incentive is for a mandatory vaccination program.

VACCINES AVAILABLE IN THE UNITED STATES

As of the publication of this book, all of the vaccines listed below are available in the United States.

Adenovirus
Anthrax
Cholera
Diphtheria
Haemophilus influenza type b
Hepatitis A
Hepatitis B
Herpes simplex virus
Influenza
Lyme disease
Japanese encephalitis
Measles

Meningococcal meningitis

Mumps

Pertussis

Plague *(Yersinia pestis)*

Pneumococcal infection

Polio

Rabies

Rotavirus

Rubella

Russian spring-summer encephalitis

Smallpox

Tetanus

Tuberculosis

Typhoid

Varicella (chicken pox)

Western equine encephalitis

Yellow fever

The following vaccines may be available soon.

Allergy and hay fever

Hepatitis C

HIV

Hypercholesterolemia

Human papillomavirus

Paramyxovirus (RSV A and B)

Salmonella typhi

Streptococcus

WHAT IS THE ROLE OF ANTIBIOTICS IN DISEASE CONTROL?

Throughout the history of medicine—and even today—physicians and consumers alike search for the magic bullet that can cure disease effortlessly, with no help from the host. Even though deep down we know this is impossible, we continue the search. Antibiotics were the first magic bullet in medicine. These bullets are intended to directly affect the pathogenic microbes, sparing harm to the host, or the diseased person. With the discovery of antibiotics, everyone thought that disease had been conquered and that we would no longer endure continuing epidemics. By 1965 physicians felt little threat from bacterial disease, and scientists were no longer interested in pursuing research on antibiotics. In 1969 the U.S. Surgeon General declared that the "war against infectious disease has been won."

We have found, however, that antibiotics are a two-edged sword. On the one hand, they attack and kill bacteria; on the other, they are not without side effects. Even though there are more antibiotics than ever available today, death caused by sepsis (bacterial infection of the blood) has increased sevenfold in U.S. hospitals in the past fifteen years. Death from infectious disease in general has risen 58 percent in the same span of time, and we are faced with new infectious diseases that we do not know how to treat. Why? Let us first examine the history of antibiotics.

The word *antibiotic* means "against life" and was originally used by the Greeks to describe resistance to the normal changes of life. Later it was used to refer to a nonbelief in life on other planets. In 1941 the American microbiologist Selman Waksman used the word to specify a substance from one microorganism that would inhibit the growth of another bacterium. Much of the pioneering work on the development of antibiotics was done by the German bacteriologist Paul Ehrlich in the early 1900s. His work indicated that there were agents that would kill some living things but not others. This concept is crucial in terms of infection because it is important to kill the infectious agent without killing the patient. Through his work, Ehrlich discovered Salvarsan (arsphenamine), a drug to treat syphilis. The term *chemotherapy* was coined by Ehrlich to refer to the selective destruction of certain cells by chemicals. This term is now applied more popularly to the treatment of cancer, where it also means the selective killing of certain cells by chemicals, in this case, tumor cells rather than bacterial cells.

Although it originally referred to a natural substance produced by one microorganism that would affect another microorganism, the term *antibiotic* is typically used today to designate a substance (synthetic or naturally occurring) that inhibits the growth of a microorganism. The first antibiotics that proved useful were the sulfa drugs, discovered by the chemist Gerhard Domagk, who worked for the Bayer Chemical Company in Germany in the 1930s. Domagk's work toward finding an effective chemotherapy was inspired by the horrors he saw at field hospitals during World War I, among them soldiers dying of staph, strep, and gangrene infections. While conducting research years later on the human immune system, he observed that damaged bacteria were destroyed by the immune system more quickly than were intact bacteria. Finally, after years of failed experiments, he found a drug that did not kill the bacteria on a petri dish, but did save the lives of mice with lethal strep infections. The drug damaged the bacterial cells, which were then destroyed more easily by the body's immune system. This work resulted in the drug known as Prontosil, a treatment for streptococcal infections. In the body, Prontosil is converted to sulfanilamide, the active ingredient. In 1939 Domagk was awarded the Nobel Prize in Physiology or Medicine for his work.

Then, in 1929, the British bacteriologist Sir Alexander Fleming noticed that a culture plate on which he was growing colonies of staphylococci was contaminated with a fungus. Most microbiologists would be disappointed because the plate had become contaminated and would simply start over. But Fleming also noticed that there were no bacteria evident around the spot where the fungus was growing. This prompted the scientist to purify the substance made by the fungus that inhibited the growth of the bacteria. Because the fungus was called *Penicillium*, he named the substance he purified from it penicillin. This serendipitous discovery paved the way for future research on antibiotics.

Because penicillin was difficult to purify and a rather unstable molecule, Fleming attracted little interest from other scientists or drug companies. During World War II, infectious disease was the leading cause of death among soldiers on the battlefield. Scientists began to seek ways to mass-produce penicillin for broad use among military personnel. Later, two other British microbiologists, Ernst Chain and Sir Howard Florey, were able to purify larger amounts of

penicillin and were finally able to convince the drug companies
Merck, Squibb, and Pfizer of its value. By the end of the war, there
was enough penicillin available to treat both soldiers and civilians.
The discovery of antibiotics was of great advantage at the time, because many people died from such diseases as pneumonia, meningitis,
and tuberculosis. In fact, antibiotics were called magic bullets because of the speed of recovery made by sick patients. Alexander
Fleming shared the Nobel Prize with Chain and Florey in 1945 for
their work on penicillin.

For the first time in history, medicine could actually cure common diseases. Antibiotics also allowed other fields of medicine, such
as surgery, to expand. Surgeries once too risky to perform became
less likely to introduce infection, owing to the use of antibiotics.
More and more antibiotics were discovered, and variations of penicillin were synthesized. These antibiotics were also a boon to the
U. S. pharmaceutical industry. Antibiotics have indeed proved useful in saving individual human lives from infectious disease. From a
public health standpoint, however, antibiotics cannot claim responsibility for eradicating any disease. Cases of scarlet fever as well as
typhoid were already in decline and at a very low level in the 1940s,
when the antibiotics penicillin and chloramphenicol began being
used to treat them. Credit for big drops in infectious disease rates
must go to public health measures, such as cleaning up the sewers.
The diseases themselves, which have normal phases of waxing and
waning, were on the wane when antibiotics were finally introduced.

HOW DO ANTIBIOTICS WORK?

Antibiotics interrupt specific aspects of the growth of bacteria—for
instance, by interfering with the formation of the cell wall. Antibiotics usually work on a biochemical pathway found in the bacteria.
There are four main ways in which antibiotics affect bacteria: They
interfere with the ability of the bacteria to make the cell wall; alter
the transport of nutrients across the bacterial cell membrane; curb
the capacity of the bacteria to make proteins; and suppress the ability of the bacteria to make nucleic acids, or DNA. By blocking one

of these steps, an antibiotic can either kill or slow down the growth of a bacterium. Even though we have more than 160 antibiotics available today, they all work in one of these four ways.

TABLE 6. THE ANTIBACTERIAL ACTION OF ANTIBIOTICS

Action	Antibiotic
Inhibits cell wall synthesis	Penicillin, vancomycin, bacitracin, cephalosporin
Inhibits cell membrane function	Amphotericin B, polymyxins, antifungals (polyenes, azoles)
Inhibits protein synthesis	Tetracyclines, streptocmycin, erythromycins, chloramphenicol
Inhibits nucleic acid, or DNA, synthesis	Sulfonamides, trimethoprim

WHAT ARE THE SIDE EFFECTS OF ANTIBIOTICS?

Antibiotics have many adverse effects on the body. Excessive use of antibiotics may cause diarrhea and loss of nutrients due to diarrhea, food allergies, allergic reactions, irritable bowel syndrome, seizures, liver damage, and immune suppression. Antibiotics do not selectively kill pathogens, but, rather, kill a variety of bacteria, and alter the ratio of bacterial species in the body by doing so. This makes the body more prone to other infections. Antibiotics also contribute to chronic fatigue syndrome. The most serious side effect, however, is antibiotic resistance, which can take a heavy toll in terms of lives and money.

There has been a proliferation of reports of antibiotic resistance in the past few years. Among these are reports of increased resistance spreading through hospitals and nursing homes. One example of this is a citywide outbreak of ceftazidime-resistant bacteria in Chicago-area nursing homes reported in 1999. Ceftazidime is a third-generation cephalosporin antibiotic used for infections caused by gram-negative rods—or enteric bacteria. It is especially useful for treating meningitis because, unlike most drugs, it has the capability of passing into the spinal fluid. Analysis of the bacterial DNA from this outbreak indicated that this resistance was not directly due to ceftazidime use but instead was probably the result of overuse of other antibiotics that supported the production of what is referred to as extended-spectrum beta-lactamases (ESBLs) in these bacteria. These ESBLs are capable of causing resistance to a broad number of related antibiotics.[10]

Resistance of *Staphylococcus aureus* to methicillin has been a long-term problem, and vancomycin has been considered the best weapon against this resistant bacterium. However, in 1999 the first report of a vancomycin-resistant *S. aureus* was reported in the United States. In 1997 the first worldwide report of vancomycin resistance occurred in Japan. This raises great concern for practitioners treating infections of this type. People particularly at risk for *S. aureus* infections are those with underlying medical conditions and those with indwelling catheters in hospital settings.[11]

Helicobacter pylori is a gram-negative rod bacterium that is sometimes found in the stomach and is associated with stomach ulcers and possibly stomach cancer. Treatment for *H. pylori* typically includes a mixture of amoxicillin with other antibiotics. However, *H. pylori* infections may become more difficult to eradicate, as antibiotic resistance recently has been found toward clarithromycin, metronidazole, and amoxicillin. These incidences appear to be related to the widespread use of these antibiotics in the community.[12] Many people, however, are found to be infected with *H. pylori* without any symptoms of disease. For this reason, some practitioners question whether asymptomatic *H. pylori* infections should be treated at all.

There is now significant resistance to the antibiotics ampicillin, cephalothin, and sulfamethoxazol in bacteria that cause urinary tract infections.[13] Penicillin-resistant *Streptococcus pneumonia*, an organism responsible for pneumonia, otitis media, and meningitis, has been a long-standing problem. A recent report showed that 52 percent of patients hospitalized for pneumococcal pneumonia had drug resistance to penicillin, cephalosporin, or a macrolid drug such as erythromycin.[14] ← This is what they gave me for pneumonia.

Mycobacterium tuberculosis, the organism responsible for tuberculosis, seems to have developed multiple-drug resistance.

Interestingly, resistance to antibiotics is nothing new and was first predicted in the 1940s shortly after the introduction of penicillin.[15] However, with widespread antibiotic use, the problem of antibiotic resistance could put the treatment of serious infectious diseases in jeopardy, and immediate action must be taken to avoid further problems.

WHAT IS ANTIBIOTIC RESISTANCE?

Bacteria have found a way to outsmart antibiotics. After being exposed to an antibiotic, they begin to produce enzymes that enable them to shield themselves from that antibiotic. This prevents the antibiotic from killing the bacteria, a mechanism of action termed antibiotic resistance. This problem has become so profound that some scientists predict that we are on the verge of a medical disaster in which small infections could turn lethal, setting back medicine to where it was in the pre-antibiotic period. The first case of bacterial resistance was seen in 1942, just a few years after clinicians began administering penicillin. Since that time, drug manufacturers have been continually modifying the chemical structure of penicillin to overcome this resistance, but the bacteria continue to mutate and become resistant to the new drugs, usually within just a few years of their introduction.

Resistance is an environmental adaptation, or evolution, that occurs through a change in the bacterial DNA. Because the alteration lies within the genetic code, it is passed on to the next generation. Bacteria are also able to trade pieces of DNA with other bacteria, allowing a gene to travel rapidly in a bacterial population. This is consistent with Darwin's "survival of the fittest" theory— if one bacterial cell in a population has the gene for penicillin resistance, when the population is exposed to penicillin, only that bacterium survives to pass on the resistant gene to the next generation, thus the next generation is fully resistant to penicillin. Scientists have recently discovered new mechanisms of DNA transfer between bacteria—transposons and integrons—which brings to light the serious nature of the problem. There is also a nongenetic origin for bacterial resistance to antibiotics. Some bacteria have the ability to become dormant under certain conditions. Antibiotics cannot kill dormant bacteria, and these dormant bacteria can thus survive antibiotic treatment. In general, we can say that a combination of the overprescription of antibiotics, the misprescription of antibiotics, and the use of antibiotics in animal husbandry are responsible for the rising incidence of antibiotic resistance.

Bacterial resistance is a grave public health concern, but what causes it? Most cases of bacterial resistance stem from overuse and misuse of antibiotics. It is estimated that in 50 to 60 percent of cases, antibiotics are not appropriate for the specific condition for which they are administered. There are several rules that should be followed for prescribing antibiotics. Antibiotics should never be taken for viral infections, such as colds and flu. They are ineffective against viruses. And they should rarely be used as prophylaxis, or to prevent an infection. Unfortunately, antibiotics are often prescribed just to pacify a patient who insists on walking away with a medicine of some kind. Needless to say, this is an inappropriate application of antibiotics. This type of use is quite common in Third World countries, where antibiotics are handed out freely at local clinics, at inappropriate doses, and without oversight by a physician. Antibiotics should also not be used to treat pain, such as dental pain.

Often, broad-spectrum antibiotics, which kill a wide variety of bacteria, are used when a narrow-spectrum type would work. This is like dropping a bomb when firing a bullet would do. Even when a narrow-spectrum antibiotic is used, it is often the wrong one. Physicians are taught in medical school to identify the organism before prescribing an antibiotic, but they seldom do so. Almost every microbiologist and drug manufacturer recommends that a culture be taken before a drug is prescribed. A culture, or a sample of the infection, can identify the infectious agent and determine which antibiotic is effective against it, but culturing takes time, and physicians usually prescribe an antibiotic based on some "knowledge" of which infectious agents are present. Antibiotics are routinely administered for sore throats that are suspected of being strep infections. If cultures were taken from these patients, the actual number that would be strep positive would be very low. At the very least a rapid test for strep antigen should be done. However, this is not as accurate as a culture. To limit the threat of bacterial resistance and maintain antibiotic effectiveness for the life-threatening conditions they were meant to treat, serious and wide-ranging change will have to take place in our society.

Antibiotic use in the agricultural industry also contributes to the overall problem of bacterial resistance. Not only are antibiotics found in animal feed; they are also used to treat some crops and are used in fish farming. The use of antibiotics in agriculture is soaring. Antibiotics in animal feed are intended to keep the animals healthy and promote growth, generating a better price at slaughter. Farmers treat their cows with antibiotics so much that a glass of milk may contain up to eighty different antibiotics. This overuse of antibiotics in beef has created the new, more toxic strain of *E. coli* that has killed many people who have eaten undercooked beef. Some outbreaks of illness caused by *E. coli* 0157:H7 have been associated with produce that came in contact with manure.[16] A new strain of bacteria, which has been identified in chickens, is resistant to the fluoroquinolone antibiotics. The possibility of these resistant strains being passed to humans is real. One study has shown that workers in the poultry industry have the same types of antibiotic-resistant *E. coli* in their digestive tracts as were found in chickens.[17] Even more convincing of the connection between antibiotic use in animals and antibiotic resistance in humans is a study reported in the *New England Journal of Medicine* in 1999. This study showed an eightfold increase in drug-resistant cases of diarrhea following the approval and use of fluoroquinolones in poultry production. The bacterium responsible for this diarrhea is *Campylobacter jejuni.* What's more, DNA fingerprinting analysis showed that the *C. jejuni* found in the human infections were the same as those found in the chickens. This documents that quinolones in animals raised as food for humans leads to the transfer of resistant and pathogenic bacteria to humans through the food chain.[18]

The Food and Drug Administration is finally revising its guidelines for antibiotic use in animals. Especially at issue is the use of antibiotics that are also used to treat human diseases. With huge pressure from both the drug and agricultural industries promoting these antibiotics, it is difficult to say how much the FDA will be able to curb the use of antibiotics in agriculture.

Antibiotics were first approved as feed additives for farm use in 1951. In 1963 antibiotic resistant bacteria were first identified in feedlots.[19] The Animal Health Institute is a U.S. trade association representing makers of animal health care products, such as vaccines, pharmaceuticals, and feed additives. The Animal Health Institute supports the use of antibiotics in feed, saying that it controls intestinal bacteria that might interfere with digestion, thus allowing the animals to grow faster and stronger than they normally would. Antibiotics are also administered at higher levels to prevent lung infections in animals. Although the Animal Health Institute contends that the danger to humans of using antibiotics in feed is negligible, this may not be the case. Statistics from the Centers for Disease Control indicate that 12 percent of *E. coli* 0157:H7 organisms and 34 percent of *Salmonella* species demonstrate antibiotic resistance.

What can you do to decrease the risk of bacterial resistance? Question your physician if he or she prescribes an antibiotic to be sure a bacterial disease is present. Question whether a more narrow-spectrum antibiotic can be used. And support farmers who don't use antibiotics.

WHAT ARE THE SIDE EFFECTS OF SPECIFIC ANTIBIOTICS?

The more personal side effects of antibiotic therapy vary with each antibiotic. Sometimes the side effects are serious enough that an antibiotic can be used only topically—gramicidin, for example. The risk of absorbing too much through the skin increases with the size of the area treated. Burn patients are often given a large dose of antibiotics, so side effects are more common among them. Polymyxin B sulfate must be applied topically with care because nerve and kidney damage can result if too much is absorbed through the skin. Many antibiotics sometimes cause dermatitis, especially neomycin.

The most widely used antibiotics are members of the penicillin family. Penicillins are typically active against gram-positive bacteria, as they interfere with production of the bacterial cell wall found in these organisms. There are some members of the penicillin family, such as amoxicillin, that are active against gram-negative bacteria. Penicillin is part of a family of antibiotics referred to as beta lactams, based on similarities in their chemical structure. Bacteria that are resistant to penicillin typically produce an enzyme that can break the beta-lactam ring of penicillin, rendering it inactive. Newer synthetic drugs based on the structure of penicillin, such as cephalosporins (for example, methicillin), are beta lactamase resistant because their chemical structure blocks the beta lactam ring, making it inaccessible to the bacterial enzyme. Many staphylococci strains are resistant to the beta-lactamase-resistant penicillins, however, because they have adapted additional mechanisms of protection.

Penicillin leaves the body through a number of paths: urine, sputum, and milk, for example. The levels present in milk from cows that have been treated with penicillin for mastitis can be a problem for humans with penicillin allergies. Penicillins are less toxic, however, than any of the other antibiotics. Allergies to penicillin have developed in many people, possibly as the result of its widespread usage. All penicillins are irritating to the central nervous system and can increase excitability. Abnormalities in sodium and potassium levels can also occur, which may affect muscles— including the heart muscle. On injection of high concentrations, some penicillins will cause irritation to the muscle or vein and accompanying pain, thrombophlebitis, or nerve degeneration. Taken orally, large amounts of penicillin can bring on nausea, vomiting, and diarrhea. Penicillin usage results in an imbalance of body flora, causing overgrowth of staphylococci, pseudomonas, *Proteus* organisms, or yeasts. In children, granulocytopenia can stem from penicillin use. Other side effects include kidney inflammation, bleeding, rashes, and decreases in potassium levels that can lead to changes in blood pH.[20]

Chloramphenicol, a broad-spectrum antibiotic that was derived in 1947 from the fungus *Streptomyces venezuelae*, is now made synthetically. It acts to block the ability of bacterial cells to make protein. This antibiotic is most often used for *Salmonella* infections (such as typhoid fever), *Haemophilus influenzae* infections (such as meningitis), and central nervous system infections. Resistant bacteria are able to inactivate the drug. Toxic effects of chloramphenicol include nausea, vomiting, diarrhea, and disturbances in red blood cell production. Aplastic anemia is a rare but fatal consequence of chloramphenicol administration. Chloramphenicol is especially toxic to infants, causing gray baby syndrome. It can also have a profound effect on the metabolism of other drugs, making them more potent. Chloramphenicol was widely overused between 1948 and 1950, when it was administered for minor respiratory complaints and resulted in many cases of aplastic anemia.[21]

The tetracyclines are another class of broad-spectrum antibiotics that are isolated from various *Streptomyces* species of fungus. The specific drug tetracycline is synthesized from another, similar antibiotic isolated from *S. aureofaciens*. Tetracyclines are active against many bacteria, both gram positive and gram negative. They act similarly to chloramphenicol by blocking the bacteria's ability to make new proteins, which are essential to life. Because human cells do not take up tetracycline as readily as bacteria do, protein synthesis is not blocked in the human. This is the type of selective toxicity that is required of an antibiotic.

Because tetracyclines are broad spectrum, they are most useful against infections caused by more than one bacterium, such as sinus infections. They are also useful against *Mycoplasma*-induced pneumonia and *Chlamydia*, *Rickettsia*, and *Vibrio* species, although many *Vibrio* species are resistant. Tetracycline is widely, and probably inappropriately, prescribed for acne, urinary tract infections, and bronchitis. Tetracycline chelates, or binds with, metals and thus should not be taken with milk (owing to the calcium content), antacids, or iron compounds, as this could cause loss of these micronutrient metals from the body. Bound to calcium, it can deposit into growing bones, causing deformities or slowed growth as well as yellowed teeth. For this reason, it is not appropriate for pregnant women or children. Tetracycline can produce sensitivity reactions, such as fever and skin rash; nausea, vomiting, and diarrhea; intestinal irritation; and anorexia. After a few days of use, the normal flora of the intestines becomes modified, allowing pseudomonads, *Proteus* organisms, staphylococci, resistant coliforms, clostridia, and *Candida* yeast to dominate. The worse-case scenario in this regard is severe enterocolitis followed by shock and then death. Liver and kidney toxicities can occur with tetracycline. It also interferes with prothrombin formation, a step in blood coagulation, resulting in bleeding. It should not be used by people with bleeding problems or those taking anticoagulant drugs— for thrombosis, for instance. Photosensitization may be a problem in fair-skinned people, and dizziness and vertigo are also possible side effects.[22]

Tetracyclines have a history of misuse for minor illnesses that has resulted in the emergence of "superbugs." These antibiotics are also widely used in animal feeds.

Vancomycin is active against gram-positive bacteria, such as staphylococci, by blocking the bacterial cell from making its cell wall. Resistance to vancomycin is rare, and it is often used against organisms that have become resistant to penicillins and methicillins. Because it is not absorbed from the intestinal tract, it must be administered intravenously, except for gastrointestinal infections, such as enterocolitis. Adverse side effects of vancomycin are not common, but they include ototoxicity (toxicity to the ear that may result in loss of hearing) and kidney toxicity as well as flushing of the face. This drug has been considered the last-chance treatment for staphylococcus infections that have developed resistance. Unfortunately, on February 8, 1999, the *New England Journal of Medicine* reported the first three cases of vancomycin-resistant *Staphylococcus aureus* infection in the United States, making these infections even more difficult to treat.[23]

There are also indirect adverse effects of antibiotics. For instance, owing to the change in types of bacteria in the intestinal tract, nutritional status can be affected, especially the intake of vitamins K, A, B_{12}, and C as well as magnesium, folic acid, and potassium. At the same time, antibiotics do save lives and have contributed to improved health care and an overall improved standard of living. The issue has two sides, the good and the bad. Only by understanding both of these sides can each person make an informed decision.

TABLE 7. SIDE EFFECTS OF ANTIBIOTICS

Common	Less common	Rare
Nausea	Seizures	Death
Vomiting	Liver damage	Acute liver injury
Diarrhea	Kidney damage	Aplastic anemia
Allergic reactions	Cardiovascular effects	Bone marrow toxicity
Skin rashes	Colitis	Lupus syndrome
Reactions with other drugs	Ear damage/deafness	Cancer
Fever	Opportunistic fungal infections	Intestinal cramps

WHEN SHOULD I SEE A DOCTOR ABOUT GETTING ANTIBIOTICS?

Antibiotics save lives and, when indicated, should be used. The problem is that they are overused and misused and not reserved for those life-threatening situations for which they were intended. If you have an infection, see your doctor to find out if bacteria are to blame. Knowing when antibiotics are called for, isn't always easy to determine, however, even for a doctor. For instance, if you have sinusitis, who knows whether the culprits are viruses or bacteria—without taking a sample from your sinus cavity? If your doctor goes for the prescription pad, ask, "Do you really think I need antibiotics?" Occasionally doctors aren't sure but suspect you want such medication. Sometimes you can take the prescription and wait to see if the illness improves on its own within a day two.

Although herbs and home remedies are useful for conditions that are not life threatening, it is important to know where to draw the line. For herbs to be effective, they should be taken at the first sign of illness.

Linda B. White, M.D., coauthor of *Kids, Herbs, and Health,* warns that children under the age of two years have less mature immune systems. They're more susceptible to bacterial infections of the blood (bacteremia) and to serious infections such as pneumonia and meningitis. Some infections, such as strep throat, can produce lifelong complications if not treated. She suggests that you call your doctor anytime your infant under six months acts sick or if your child under two years old runs a fever over 102ºF (38.8ºC). Otherwise, gentle herbs make great allies against common childhood illnesses. They can boost immunity, fight infection, and alleviate symptoms. Just know that in order for them to work most effectively, you need to start early in the course of the illness and give appropriate doses at frequent intervals. A qualified herbal practitioner can help guide you. A good rule of thumb for calling your doctor is do so when the child is clearly very ill, symptoms worsen, or symptoms fail to improve markedly within three days of the start of home treatment.

It is always good to have the support of an understanding physician if you have an infectious disease. The purpose of this book is to help you understand when it is appropriate and when it is not appropriate to take antibiotics.

ANTIFUNGAL AGENTS

Antibacterial drugs rarely work to kill a fungus. Specific antifungal agents are needed for this, and even so, fungal infections are difficult to treat because fungi can form spores that remain dormant for long periods. In spite of the difficulty of administering it and the range of side effects, amphotericin B, which is produced by *Streptomyces noduosus,* is the most effective antibiotic drug for treating severe and widespread fungal infection. Amphotericin and related polyene antibiotics act by attacking the fungal cell membrane, which is composed of lipids different from those of bacterial or human cell membranes. Organisms can develop resistance to amphotericin by changing the composition of their membranes. Amphotericin B is not well absorbed in the gastrointestinal tract and thus is generally given by intravenous injection rather than orally. Amphotericin B usually causes chills, fever, vomiting, and headache. Less often there is kidney and liver damage, followed by decreased blood pressure, an imbalance in blood ions, and neurological symptoms.[24]

Another group of antifungal antibiotics are the azoles, which include clotrimazole, miconazole, and ketoconazole. They are completely synthetic drugs, not derived from other fungal or bacterial species. These drugs block the production of a lipid, ergosterol, found in the fungal cell membrane. The way in which the azoles thwart lipid synthesis is by blocking an enzyme that is also found in the liver and is involved in the detoxification of many drugs and toxins—cytochrome P450. Many of the azoles are used only on the skin, but some are administered orally and affect human cytochrome P450 enzymes. These effects can inhibit the production of some of the steroid hormones and affect the concentrations of other drugs that are taken simultaneously. Adverse effects of these antibiotics include vomiting, high blood lipid levels, altered blood electrolyte levels, skin rashes, liver damage, blood clots, and other blood disorders. Many of this class of antibiotics are used topically for yeast infections with little fear of side effects. Miconazole is the preferred drug for vaginal yeast infections. Care must be taken even in applying the drug topically, however; some of the drug is absorbed through the skin and can enter the bloodstream.[25]

Nystatin is an antifungal agent often found in over-the-counter creams in combination with other antibiotics. It is meant to be applied routinely on the skin for cuts and scrapes. It is also used topically or orally for candida (yeast) infections. It is safer than many antibiotics, and few side effects have been reported for this agent other than allergic skin reactions.[26]

A Personal Account

At a friend's house one day, Marilyn's daughter, Linda, got a small bug bite. With good intentions, the friend's mother applied an over-the-counter fungal cream to the bite to keep it from becoming infected. Unfortunately, Linda had a severe allergic reaction to the cream. Initially, her skin became inflamed and sore, but then the reaction spread through her body. She suffered open sores all over, even on her eyelids. Because her immune system was preoccupied with the allergic reaction, she developed an opportunistic infection—Epstein-Barr virus. (This agent is the same virus that causes mononucleosis.) Although Marilyn was able to treat her daughter's sores with tea tree oil and chamomile, Linda remained practically bedridden for six months. Even eight years later, she suffers from chronic fatigue syndrome, possibly the result of her reaction to the antifungal drug.

ANTIVIRAL AGENTS

Viral growth depends on the host cell's DNA, RNA, and protein synthesis pathways. Viruses are intracellular parasites; when they enter a cell, they tend to take over its normal processes. For this reason, it has been most difficult to develop drugs to prevent their growth without inhibiting the growth of normal cells. The growth of viral particles reaches its peak about the same time as clinical symptoms first appear, which also makes treatment difficult. Injection of a class of immunoglobulins called gamma globulins, taken from donor blood during the early part of infection, can be effective in decreasing the seriousness of the disease. This treatment is often undertaken if one is exposed to hepatitis or rabies, for example.

Acyclovir is one of a family of drugs that are similar in chemical structure to the bases that make up DNA and RNA and can inhibit the manufacture of new DNA. In large doses, it can even inhibit the synthesis of new human DNA. Developed in the 1970s, it is used primarily as a topical agent for treating herpes infections, such as cold sores, genital warts, and shingles; intravenously it can treat more serious conditions. It is recommended that acyclovir be used with care, to minimize the development of the resistant strains of herpes that arise from overuse of the drug. The side effects of topical acyclovir include itching, mild pain, and some stinging. Because of its wide use, we are now seeing acyclovir-resistant herpesviruses.[27, 28]

In a new class of useful antiviral drugs are the interferons. As mentioned previously, these are proteins produced by certain white blood cells as well as other cell types called fibroblasts to inhibit viral growth in the body. Interferons have proved to be effective in treating some viral infections as well as certain types of cancer, but they have quite a few side effects, including fever, fatigue, headaches, weakness, myalgia, anemia, gastrointestinal problems, and cardiovascular disturbances.[29]

In the past few years many potential antiviral drugs have been introduced, including the anti-AIDS drug AZT. The jury is still out on the effectiveness and side effects of these drugs. Newer antiviral drugs used to treat influenza include the neuraminidase inhibitors oseltamivir (Tamiflu) and zanamivir (Relenza). Side effects include nausea, vomiting, bronchitis, and sleep disturbances.

INFECTION-CONTROL PROGRAMS

At one time, women frequently died from infections of the uterus after giving birth. This trend finally declined when it was realized that physicians were going directly from performing autopsies in the morgue to attending childbirth, carrying with them infectious agents from the corpses. The solution was simple—physicians needed to wash their hands between the morgue and the delivery room. Today, surgeons scrub before entering the operating room to avoid introducing bacteria into their patients.

Hospitals and health care facilities have in place infection-control programs to minimize the risk of spreading infections from one person to another. Infectious diseases are spread in a number of ways—by human-to-human contact, by animal-to-human contact, by human contact with an infected surface, through tiny droplets of infectious agents suspended in the air, and by a common vehicle such as food or water. Even with preventive measures, a hospital can be a dangerous place to be. As many as 5 percent of all patients will acquire infections while they are in the hospital. Most of these infections are due to *Staphylococcus* organisms. These are called nosocomial infections, and they can increase time spent in the hospital as well as cause death, in some cases. Hospital patients often have a weakened immune system owing to their disease or to treatments given to them in the hospital. A weakened immune system can make a patient more susceptible to secondary infection. Add this to such procedures as surgery that can introduce infectious agents into the patient and contact with other patients, workers, or visitors carrying infectious disease, and you will understand the dangers.

Because the risk of spreading infections is so great in a hospital, many precautions are taken. Health care workers routinely wear gloves whether or not a patient has an infection, and patients who have a known contagious disease are isolated. Any hospital worker who comes in contact with an infected person wears gloves and a gown to minimize the risk of carrying the infectious agent into other areas. Equipment used in a room where a patient is isolated is decontaminated before reuse. All patients who are immuno-compromised are put in protective isolation to lower the risk that infectious agents brought into their room will infect them. Any hospital worker with an infection—even a cold—is restricted from entering isolation rooms. In addition, hospital workers are periodically tested to determine if they are carriers of antibiotic-resistant *Staphylococcus aureus,* as infections caused by this organism are the most common hospital-acquired contagions. Special care is also taken with hospital ventilation systems, to prevent recirculation of contaminated air carrying infectious particles.

Infection-control guidelines are just as important in nursing homes, clinics, child-care centers, restaurants, and the home. To prevent the spread of infectious disease through a community, such agencies as the Centers for Disease Control have made certain recommendations. These precautions include vaccination against diseases, frequent washing of hands, thorough cooking of food, careful and directed use of antibiotics, visits to the doctor for infections that do not heal, avoidance of areas with a lot of insects, caution around unfamiliar animals, avoidance of unprotected sex or intravenous drug use, and safeguards against infectious diseases when traveling. Possibly the most important of these recommendations is to wash the hands often. Sanitation and hygiene have been shown repeatedly to lower disease risks.

There are ways that you can curtail the spread of disease in your home and workplace. First, boost your immunity. A strong immune system will make it less likely for an infectious agent to invade your body. Stay healthy with a good diet and exercise. The importance of good, wholesome foods and physical activity cannot be overemphasized. There are also herbs to promote immunity that can be taken at the first sign of illness, such as echinacea *(Echinacea angustifolia)*. Other herbs with antibiotic properties can be applied topically on skin wounds in the place of antibiotic creams—for example, goldenseal *(Hydrastis canadensis)* and tea tree oil *(Melaleuca alternifolia)*. In the form of essential oils, some herbs can be used in diffusers or diluted in water to be dispersed through a room where someone has been sick; this will decrease the risk of airborne transmission of infectious agents. Tea tree oil, rosemary *(Rosmarinus officinalis)*, and eucalyptus *(Eucalyptus radiata)* are commonly used for this purpose. (*See* chapter 8 for more specific information on herbs.)

Diseases invariably accompany poor sanitation, making epidemics prevalent in developing countries. Clean water and reliable sewage systems are essential for good hygiene. The single most important way to stop the spread of infection is to wash your hands. Antibiotic soaps are not necessary for this purpose and may even be harmful, both by irritating the skin and by promoting bacterial resistance. To wash your hands, lather them well for thirty seconds and rinse with warm water. This will remove most of the harmful bacteria from your hands. Then use a lotion to keep the skin from drying out and cracking. This will also prevent bacteria from entering the skin.

Disinfectants and Antiseptics

Disinfectants and antiseptics are antibacterial agents that are applied to surfaces to kill infectious agents. They differ from antibiotics in that they are often toxic to the host and cannot be taken internally or sometimes even touch the skin. Nevertheless, they are important to use to kill germs that live on surfaces (doorknobs and countertops, for example) in your house. Disinfectants sometimes include phenol compounds, formaldehyde, glutaraldehyde, bleach, and quaternary ammonium compounds. Silver is one disinfectant that is safe to use on the skin, and it can be found in some topical ointments. There are also many natural disinfectants, among them essential oils distilled from herbs.[30] Put a few drops of essential oil in a mister with water. Spray this solution on doorknobs, bedding, bathroom faucets, keyboards, countertops, and anywhere an infectious person might sneeze.

Essential oils with
antiseptic/antimicrobial activity

Basil *(Ocimum basilicum)*
Bay *(Pimenta racemosa)*
Benzoin *(Styrax benzoin dryander)*
Bergamot *(Citrus aurantium)*
Black pepper *(Piper nigrum)*
Cardamom *(Elettaria cardamomum maton)*
Cedarwood *(Cedrus atlantica)*
Chamomile, German *(Matricaria recutita)*
Chamomile, Roman *(Chamaemelum nobile)*
Cinnamon *(Cinnamomum zeylanicum)*
Clary sage *(Salvia sclarea)*
Clove *(Syzygium aromaticum)*
Eucalyptus *(Eucalyptus citriodora, E. globulus, E. radiata)*

Fennel *(Foeniculum vulgare)*
Frankincense *(Boswellia carterii)*
Geranium (*Pelargonium* spp.)
Grapefruit *(Citrus paradisi)*
Juniper *(Juniperus communis)*
Lavender *(Lavandula angustifolia)*
Lemon *(Citrus limonum)*
Marigold, Pot *(Calendula officinalis)*
Marjoram *(Origanum majorana)*
Melissa *(Melissa officinalis)*
Myrrh *(Commiphora myrrha)*
Neroli *(Citrus aurantium)*
Orange *(Citrus aurantium)*
Oregano *(Origanum vulgare)*
Patchouli *(Pogostemon cablin)*
Peppermint *(Mentha piperita)*
Pine *(Pinus sylvestris)*
Rosemary *(Rosmarinus officinalis)*
Sandalwood *(Santalum album)*
Spikenard *(Nardostachys jatamansi)*
Tea tree (*Melaleuca alternifolia*)
Thyme *(Thymus vulgaris)*
Ylang-ylang *(Canangium odorata)*

4 Does Stress Influence Health?

Have you noticed that when you are under the most stress, you tend to get sick more often—when you have the least time to stop what you are doing and rest? Scientists are learning more each day about how stress affects the body and the immune system. It is, in fact, the body's response to stress—how we handle it—that is important. Among the many ways to improve the body's reaction to stress, you can take particular herbs called adaptogens. There are also herbs that can help with specific symptoms of stress, herbs with calming or sedative effects.

Any stimulus that evokes the stress response is termed a stressor. A stressor affects the body, putting it out of balance or disrupting what is called homeostasis. The stress response helps right that imbalance. Stressors can be external or internal (psychological). Stress is an important response that evolved as a means of aiding the body in times of emergency. There are three stages to the stress response: the alarm response, the delayed response, and finally exhaustion.

The organs in the body most affected by stress are the adrenal glands. These glands are located above the kidneys and are functionally linked to the nervous system. The adrenal medulla secretes epinephrine and norepinephrine into the bloodstream in response to stress. These two hormones, or neurotransmitters, are referred to as catecholamines, and they are important in the stress response. The delayed response, or the resistance reaction, to stress is the second stage. Another section of the adrenal glands, the adrenal cortex, secretes two other classes of hormones, known as mineralocorticoids and glucocorticoids, at this stage of the body's response.

TABLE 8. TYPES OF STRESS

External, or physical, stress	Internal, or psychological, stress
Bleeding	Death of a spouse
Cold/heat	Demands of work or school
Infection	Marital conflict
Noise	Money matters
Pollution	Recalling a confrontation
Surgery	Dealing with an emergency

WHAT IS THE ALARM REACTION?

The alarm reaction, also referred to as the fight-or-flight response, evolved to help the body deal with an impending emergency by increasing physical activity. Its purpose is to give the body a short burst of energy to either fight an enemy or run from it. This was important to prehistoric people who might have encountered a saber-toothed tiger, for example, and needed to run as fast as possible to escape. It is just as important now to save a child from the path of a speeding car.

The body is able to increase its physical activity by increasing blood flow to the skeletal muscles and the brain. In doing so, the "nonessential activities" such as digestion, urination, and reproduction are shut down. The body does not need to waste its energy supplying blood to aid these processes in times of emergency.

This alarm response is initiated by nerve impulses from the brain. These nerve impulses reach the adrenal medulla gland, which then secretes epinephrine and norepinephrine into the blood. These hormones circulate through the body to stimulate the appropriate nerves. Stimulation by epinephrine and norepinephrine on nerve endings throughout the body results in a variety of physical responses including increased heart rate, blood pressure, breathing, and sweating; rerouting of blood flow from digestion to the muscles; and release of stored sugars from the liver. This short burst of epinephrine also enhances memory. This may be a way of conditioned learning to prevent someone from making the same mistake twice.

Another hormone released is enkephalin. This hormone temporarily blocks pain sensations. The result of all this is to increase a person's strength, which enables him to deal with an immediate threat in an appropriate way. We have all heard of grand feats accomplished by people under stress that range from lifting cars to performing well in a concert. A little stress, then, is a good thing. It's when stress becomes continual that it can harm the body.

WHAT IS THE RESISTANCE REACTION?

The second stage of stress is activated when the alarm reaction is not sufficient to remove the stressor imposed on the body. The cortex portion of the adrenal gland secretes additional hormones— the glucocorticoids and the mineralocorticoids—during this stage of response.

The main glucocorticoid, cortisol, ensures the presence of an adequate level of blood glucose, which is necessary to keep the muscles and the brain running. Cortisol also reduces inflammation and depresses the immune system. These two actions are necessary to allow for wound healing, but when cortisol persists under extended periods of increased stress, the results are not beneficial. Cortisol may also have a negative effect on bone tissue and thus exacerbate osteoporosis when it is administered over a long period. Another negative effect of cortisol is that it can cause an alteration of sensory perception and emotion.

Mineralocorticoids, such as aldosterone, secreted in response to stress, cause the kidneys to retain sodium ions, resulting in water retention. Water retention has two purposes: to maintain the increased blood pressure produced in the alarm reaction and to replace the volume of any blood lost. Aldosterone also induces the kidneys to eliminate hydrogen ions, which in turn increases the pH of the blood, making it more alkaline.

Other hormones that help our bodies get through a period of stress include thyroxine from the thyroid gland and growth hormone and prolactin from the pituitary gland. Together these hormones assure the cells of the body an increased energy supply in the form of the nucleotide adenosine triphosphate. This energy is necessary to support the increase in metabolism produced by the stress response.

WHAT IS EXHAUSTION?

Chronic or severe stressors may not be controlled by either the alarm response or the resistance reaction, and exhaustion may set in. This happens when hormones become depleted and energy supplies dwindle. This situation can have many consequences on the body that result in such diseases as gastritis, ulcers, arthritis, headaches, anxiety, and depression. People who experience a lot of stress may also suffer chronic disease and early death. Perhaps most shocking is that stress can cause deterioration of parts of the brain that leads not only to a decrease in learning ability and memory but also to cognitive declines associated with aging.[1]

How someone deals with stress varies with personality and physiological endowment. The types of things that cause chronic stress vary during different times of life as well. A young child may experience chronic stress in relationship to school, whereas a middle-aged person may experience it from a changing marital relationship. Stress can lead to depression or cause someone to engage in unhealthy behavior such as extramarital relationships or drinking.

There is a connection among the nervous, endocrine, and immune systems of the body that can be disrupted by stress. When this balance is disrupted, the immune system can be affected in such as way that chronic infection results. Both the humoral and the cellular immune systems are influenced by stress. Science has documented that stress can affect the progression of tuberculosis infection and herpes infection and increase the risk of infection with a cold virus.[2] Severe stress is also associated with a more rapid progression of AIDS by diminishing immunity.[3]

Other studies have shown that chronic stress can decrease the effectiveness of vaccination. When people who were experiencing stress from caring for a relative with Alzheimer's disease received an influenza vaccine, their antibody response was fourfold lower than that of people not under stress. Similar results were obtained from a study of medical students injected with hepatitis B vaccine. Those patients with lower levels of anxiety and stress had more pronounced antibody responses to the vaccination.[4] It seems that just when you need the protection of a vaccine the most, it is least effective.

THE EFFECTS OF CORTISOL ON IMMUNITY

These changes in the immune system are due mainly to elevations in cortisol and other hormones, but not to that alone. Studies in animals have shown that stress also activates a part of the brain called the periaqueductal gray area. This area is responsible for behavior and mediating immune suppression. Increases in cortisol levels are also associated with depression.

Besides having specific effects on the immune system, cortisol affects other parts of the body as well. Cortisol increases the breakdown of protein to form glucose. This causes the muscles to become very weak. The amount of protein made in the cells is also decreased, which affects the function of each specific tissue. In the case of lymphoid tissue, it prevents the production of antibodies and cytokines, which then suppresses immunity. Cortisol also alters metabolism of fats, proteins, and carbohydrates. This change in metabolism is designed to keep blood glucose levels high in order to provide energy, but it causes what is known as adrenal diabetes.

The effect of cortisol on the immune system is so profound that it is used clinically to suppress immunity. For instance, in the case of organ transplants, cortisol can prevent rejection. In cases of severe inflammation, such as arthritis, cortisol can decrease the inflammation. However, large doses of cortisol can depress the immune system to the point where it leads to fulminating infection that results in death.

Cortisol affects the immune system in the following ways:

- Decreases migration of white blood cells to areas of inflammation
- Decreases phagocytosis
- Decreases formation of prostaglandins
- Diminishes reproduction of white blood cells
- Reduces release of interleukin-1
- Reduces fever

HOW CAN YOU CONTROL STRESS?

It is important to find ways to deal with stress to limit its negative effects on the body and prevent total exhaustion. Although the way in which we react to stress is determined in part by our genetic makeup, we can exert some control. You might make changes in lifestyle including increasing social relationships by joining social or spiritual groups or talking more with supportive friends. For severe cases of stress, professional help in the form of psychological counseling may help. Through counseling, patients can change their perspective on life and thus their feelings, which in turn can decrease stress and favorably influence the immune system.

Exercise can have a positive effect on the immune system. During exercise, endorphins are released into the blood. These hormones not only provide a feeling of well-being, but also enhance the immune system and provide an analgesic effect. Many people find exercise to be of great importance in relieving stress.

A Personal Account

Elisha had been feeling unwell for some time.
She had frequent colds, was tired, and felt anxious.
She had seen a doctor but no diagnosis was made.
After reading Dr. Larry Dossey's book *Healing Words*
and learning that the power of prayer in healing had
actually been scientifically documented, she decided
it was worth a try. She purchased a book of devotions
at a bookstore and set aside fifteen minutes each day
to read from the book and meditate. Soon she was
feeling less anxious, healthier, and more energetic.
Knowing that it was her connection to God and the
spiritual realm that helped her, she continues to pray
daily, often experimenting with various types of
prayer including song and movement.

The stress hormones epinephrine and norepinephrine are made
in the body from the amino acid tyrosine. A related neurotransmitter
is serotonin, which is made from tryptophan. Low levels of serotonin
can lead to depression and anxiety. Make sure you ingest foods high in
tyrosine and tryptophan when you are under stress. Tryptophan can be
found in high-protein foods such as cheese, eggs, meat, sesame seeds,
and sunflower seeds. Tyrosine can be found in whole grains, wheat
germ, meat, seafood, peanut butter, and legumes, especially kidney beans.

The B vitamins can also be useful when you are under stress.
Most of the B vitamins are important in metabolism and energy
regulation. Pyridoxal phosphate, one of the B vitamins, is involved
in biochemical reactions, specifically one that converts tryptophan
to serotonin. Tryptophan won't help elevate serotonin levels without vitamin B around. Bitamin B_{12} has a special role in the nervous
system. Taking a supplemental B vitamin may also help your body
when you are experiencing stress. Vitamin C, too, appears to have
stress-reducing abilities. A recent study in laboratory rats showed

that those taking vitamin C produced less cortisol in response to stress than did rats not taking vitamin C.[5]

Exercises that promote relaxation are also beneficial. Try visualization, meditation, physical exercise, yoga, massage, going to bed early, painting, and diaphragmatic or rhythmic breathing. Many people find that one activity or technique suits them best.

HERBS FOR STRESS RELIEF

Some herbs help strengthen the adrenal glands to minimize exhaustion during time of stress. These herbs are called adaptogens, or restoratives, and they affect several organs of the body. Using one of these may decrease the body's negative response to stress. From a scientific perspective, it is not quite clear how these herbs work.

The herbalist Steven Foster offers these suggestions for how adaptogens might work: They alter the body's metabolism to provide more energy, they provide antioxidants that can lower the levels of toxic metabolites in the body, and they affect the hormones involved in the general adaptation to stress.[6]

Here are some adaptogens you might consider during times of great stress. Keep in mind that in most cases, these uses are based on tradition rather than science (except where indicated). This doesn't mean that they don't work; it just means that clinical scientists haven't gotten around to studying them.

Licorice *(Glycyrrhiza glabra)* is widely used as a flavoring and a sweetener, and traditionally it has been used to nourish the adrenal glands. Licorice is also anti-inflammatory and antibacterial and is used as a treatment for bronchitis and viral infections. The herbalist Christopher Hobbs suggests using 3–5 grams of licorice per day, taken in three doses either added to milk or brewed as a tea.[7] Licorice contains potentially harmful compounds, including glycyrrhizin, that affect steroid hormone activity, including the activity of corticosteroids, mineralocorticoids, and estrogen, sometimes causing water retention and increased blood pressure. Deglycyrrhizinated licorice (DGL), which has had the glycyrrhizin removed, is available and won't produce these side effects. Although deglycyrrhizinated licorice may be effective for treating ulcers it is the very hormonelike actions of glycyrrhizin that make it effective as an adaptogen.[8] Glycyrrhizin is also responsible for many of the antiviral and antibacterial properties of licorice. Nevertheless, the flavonoids found in DGL do provide some antimicrobial activity. Because of the potentially serious side effects of licorice, it is best taken under the supervision of a qualified herbalist or other health practitioner. People at most risk are those with high blood pressure and cardiac disease.

Siberian ginseng *(Eleutherococcus senticosus)* is a folk medicine from Russia that has been used for a number of conditions, including stress, depression, fatigue, and nervous breakdown. It is said to have adaptogenic effects and to increase the body's resistance to stress, although most of the scientific documentation of these effects is in the Russian literature. Siberian ginseng has also been shown to stimulate the immune system and to protect the body against some toxins. In animal studies, ginseng has shown a beneficial effect on stress.[9] Because ginseng can have a number of effects on various organ systems, it should not be taken with prescription drugs without the supervision of a physician aware of drug/herb interactions. The Russian literature suggests that it not be taken by healthy people under the age of forty, except in very small amounts, and it should not be taken over the long term. It is recommended only for a temporary boost when needed, rather than for regular usage.

American ginseng *(Panax quinquefolius)* and Korean, or Asian, ginseng *(Panax ginseng)* have certain chemicals in common and probably produce similar effects. The early medical literature did not distinguish which ginseng was being used, so confusion exists. Asian ginseng has a long history of use in Chinese medicine as a tonic or adaptogen and to improve physical strength. Although both forms of ginseng have been used as an aphrodisiac, their more important application may be in the treatment of fatigue and anxiety. Studies have shown that ginseng can improve both physical endurance and mental abilities.[10] In Germany, ginseng is labeled as a therapy for fatigue, with a suggested dose of 1–2 grams of dried root daily. As with Siberian ginseng, it should not be taken with other drugs, es-

pecially stimulants, antipsychotics, and hormones. It is contraindi-
cated for patients with cardiac disorders, diabetes, and those with
either high or low blood pressure.

Schizandra *(Schizandra chinensis)* is widely used in traditional
Chinese medicine as an adaptogen to build up the body's resistance
and improve physiological processes. It is said to increase energy
and strength.[11] Modern research indicates that it may have benefits
as a liver protector[12] and in treating HIV-1 infections.[13] It may also
improve learning. The medicinal properties of schizandra lie in the
fruit, and the suggested dose is 400–450 milligrams three times daily
in capsule or tablet form. Large doses may cause restlessness, insomnia, and labored breathing. Some writings indicate that it should
not be taken by people with epilepsy, severe hypertension, or "high
acidity," as described in Chinese medicine.

Ashwagandha *(Withania somnifera)* is a rejuvenating tonic used
in ayurvedic medicine, the folk medicine of India, and is sometimes
called Indian ginseng. Ashwagandha is said to enhance the body's
resistance to stress and depression while bolstering physical stamina.[14]
This herb also has anti-inflammatory activity. It was recently shown
to improve survival rates of mice infected with *Aspergillus* fungi.[15]
The root is used to make a decoction that is taken daily.

Reishi *(Ganoderma lucidum)* is a mushroom rather than an herb
and is commonly used in Japan. In traditional Chinese medicine,
this fungus is administered as an adaptogenic agent to help people
recover quickly from disease or to prevent disease. Reishi also enhances the immune system.[16] Use reishi in capsule or tablet form at
a dosage of 1–5 grams daily.

Gotu kola *(Centella asiatica),* or Indian pennywort, is much better
known as a wound healer than as an adaptogen, but it is traditionally used to improve the cognitive function of the brain and for help
with nervous disorders. It is also used for treating minor skin problems and varicose veins. Gotu kola has been shown to have a slight
sedative effect. Large amounts of the herb, however, can cause a
narcotic stupor, headache, and sometimes coma.[17] Extracts of the
herb have reduced the incidence of stomach ulcers in rats exposed to

stress.[18] Drink gotu kola tea made from the leaves of the herb one to three times per day or use in a tincture.

RELIEVING STRESS WITH AROMATHERAPY

Aromatherapy relieves stress through your sense of smell. Smells have a strong impact on how we feel and can play an important role in reducing stress as well as in easing depression. In her book *Essential Aromatherapy*, Susan Wormwood suggests the following essential oils for relieving stress: basil, benzoin, bergamot, carnation, Roman chamomile, clary sage, clove, frankincense, geranium, hyacinth, jasmine, lavender, lemon, linden blossom, litsea cubela (May-Chang oil), mandarin, marjoram, melissa, neroli, ormenis flower, palmarosa, patchouli, petitgrain, rose maroc, rose otto, sandalwood, vetiver, ylang-ylang, and yuzu.[19] You can see that the choices are many, so pick a scent that speaks to you. Among the most effective of these are basil, lavender, and marjoram. In his book *The Practice of Aromatherapy*, Jean Valnet also suggests cypress and rosemary. Another study showed that inhalation of lavender oil decreased the number of convulsions experienced by rats treated with electroshock or drugs that induce convulsions.[20]

Again, few studies have been performed to verify the effects of essential oils on stress. Recently, however, extracts from holy basil *(Ocimum sanctum)* were found to exhibit antistress activity by reducing the levels of corticosteroids released in rats exposed to stress.[21]

You can use essential oils as destressors in a number of ways. The easiest way is to put a few drops of your favorite essential oil on some cotton balls and place them in a plastic bag. Keep this bag with you and smell it every so often when needed. You can also add your favorite scent to a mister bottle of water and use it to spray a room. There are many types of diffusers or candles available that you can use to disperse the essential oils throughout a room as well. Perhaps the most relaxing way, though, is to use them in a warm bath. After the bath is filled, shake a few drops of the oil of your choice into the water, step in, and enjoy. Careful, though, as some essential oils can be irritating to the skin. Do not apply basil, bergamot, or lemon oils directly to the skin; in fact, basil is not a good choice to use topically at all. Save it for use in a diffuser. Oils that should not be used during pregnancy include basil, clary sage, clove, and rosemary.

CAN YOU RELIEVE OTHER SYMPTOMS OF STRESS?

There are additional herbs that may help you deal with specific symptoms of stress, such as anxiety, nervousness, and sleeplessness. These herbs can promote relaxation, pain relief, and restful sleep, possibly providing enough relief to overcome a short period of stress.

The California poppy *(Eschscholzia californica)* has legal protection as the state flower of California. This herb contains alkaloids that have sedative and anti-anxiety properties. Although it is similar to the opium poppy, it is not narcotic. Herbalists use this poppy to relieve muscle spasms that accompany stress. Use the California poppy as a tea two or three times a day or in a tincture. All parts of the plant can be used.[22]

Catnip *(Nepeta cataria)* can be grown abundantly almost anywhere. It is referred to as a calmative and is used to quiet the nervous system and relieve headaches, to calm the body, and to promote sleep. It can also be added to a bath to soothe sore muscles. Catnip is usually drunk as a tea two or three times per day, but it is also available as a tincture. Use the newly formed leaves and tips.[23]

German chamomile *(Matricaria recutita)* and Roman chamomile *(Chamaemelum nobile)* have similar effects and are often (and correctly) used interchangeably. However, Roman chamomile appears to be more strongly sedative; German chamomile appears to have stronger anti-inflammatory activity. Chamomile is widely used as a relaxant or sedative, as it can calm restlessness and tension, in addition to soothing the digestive tract. It is thought to be an especially good herb for children. Many of the effects of chamomile have been scientifically documented. One study indicates that a flavonoid from chamomile called apigenin may act similarly to the sedative class of drugs known as the benzodiazepines.[24, 25, 26] Drink chamomile as a tea one to four times a day, or as needed. The essential oil of chamomile, used in a massage oil, has been shown to improve mood and quality of life in cancer patients.[27] It may work for you, too! Many people have allergies to chamomile and to the family of plants to which it belongs. Discontinue use if any adverse effects arise. The fresh flower heads tend to lose their potency after two years.[28]

Hops *(Humulus lupulus)* is primarily thought of as an ingredient for beer, but it has historical use as a treatment for neuralgia, insomnia, nervous tension, and excitability. It acts as a sedative to promote sleep.[29] Hops can be used in several ways. Drink a beer with a high hop content (in moderation, of course), drink tea made from the flower heads of hops two or three times a day, take a tincture, or put dried hop flowers in a pouch in your pillowcase. Smelling the hops at night in your pillowcase may help promote sleep.

Kava *(Piper methysticum)*, common in the Pacific islands, is used as a sedative, anticonvulsant, anxiolytic, and muscle relaxant with slight narcotic effects. It can help relieve general tension and promote a feeling of well-being. Large doses should be avoided, as over-sedation can occur. Drink a tea made from the root of kava one to three times a day or use in a tincture equivalent to 100 milligrams of kavalactones per day.[30, 31] Do not take kava with alcohol or other antidepressants.

Lavender *(Lavandula officinalis)* has a smell that by itself can bring relaxation and pleasant memories. It is used as a sedative, relaxant, and antispasmodic. One study showed that lavender aroma increased drowsiness, improved mood, and helped volunteers perform math computations better![32] Intensive-care patients who were treated with lavender reported an improvement in mood and decreased levels of anxiety.[33] Try rubbing lavender oil on your temples to treat a headache. As an essential oil, lavender can be added to soaps, lotions, and to a warm bath, or sprinkle a few drops on a pillow at bedtime. Lavender can also be used by putting dried flowers and leaves in a sleep pillow. Although lavender tea tastes rather astringent, try lavender lemonade *(see* chapter 9) or lavender buds in sugar cookies.

Lemon balm *(Melissa officinalis)* has a wonderful lemon smell and can be used as a gentle sedative to calm nervous tension and headaches. The essential oil can be used for aromatherapy or in the bath. Drink it one to three times daily as a tea prepared from the leaves of the plant. It can also be used in a sleep pillow to promote a restful night.[34]

Passionflower *(Passiflora incarnata)* is so named because its flower symbolizes the crucifixion of Christ. The flowers of this plant contain alkaloids that are slightly narcotic and can depress the nervous system. Passionflower has been documented to have sedative properties. It can be used to treat tension, fatigue, insomnia, muscle spasms, and anxiety. It is suitable for adults as well as children. Drink it as a tea one to three times daily, using the leaves and flowers, or take as a tincture.[35, 36]

Skullcap *(Scutellaria laterifloria)* has a history of use for hysteria, nervous tension, and as a sedative. Although commonly used by herbalists to treat anxiety, it has not yet gained the attention of scientists, so there is little to no documentation of its effects. There are very few side effects noted for skullcap, but there is some indication that liver damage could be a possibility. It should not be taken by pregnant women. Take skullcap as a tea, one-half cup, three or four times daily, or as a tincture.[37, 38]

Valerian *(Valeriana officinalis)* is an antispasmodic and anxiolytic that can help promote sleep and relieve intestinal spasms. Although it smells somewhat unpleasant, the root contains compounds called valepotriates that can increase the effect of GABA (gamma amino butyric acid) in the brain. Increased GABA is associated with a sedative effect. Valerian's use as a sedative has given it the nickmane "nature's Valium." Drink valerian as a tea, one cup at a time, or use in a tincture.[39]

Wild lettuce *(Lactuca virosa)* is a mild sedative that can help alleviate insomnia and nervousness. This herb contains narcotic-like substances and has been used to dilute opium. It can also be beneficial for mild pain. Use wild lettuce in the form of a tincture.[40]

Wild oat *(Avena sativa)* is a tall grass that grows wild. It has been used throughout history as a restorative for nervous or psychological exhaustion. It can be taken over the long term for stress and a generally weak nervous system. The mild sedative action helps as a sleep aid for insomnia. Drink it as a tea three times daily or use it as a tincture.[41]

WHAT PUTS YOU AT RISK OF LOWERED IMMUNITY?

The following lifestyle choices, environmental factors, and physical conditions are all risk factors that can predispose a compromised immune system.

- Excessive drug or alcohol usage
- Excessive intestinal growth of yeast
- Excessive sugar intake
- Exposure to environmental toxins and air pollution
- Exposure to heavy metals
- Food intolerance
- Intestinal parasites
- Lack of excercise
- Lack of sleep
- Low thyroid function
- Nutrient deficiencies
- Poor hygiene
- Smoking
- Unresolved stress

5 HERBAL MEDICINE

WHY USE HERBS FOR MEDICINE?

Modern medicine has seen many advances in technology during the past twenty years. This technology has contributed to great gains in diagnosing a number of illnesses, especially cancer. It has also benefited the treatment of trauma victims who need emergency treatment. It is doubtful, however, that many gains have been made in the treatment of chronic diseases, and although antibiotics have proved to be valuable tools for treating infectious diseases, resistant strains of bacteria engendered by their overuse threaten to set us back to the time before we had antibiotics at our disposal. Medical care in the United States has also become the most expensive in the world. It is probably for these reasons that herbal medicine has seen a renaissance in recent years. People with chronic illnesses are seeking alternatives with fewer side effects. In fact, a recent survey has shown that alternative medicine has a growing presence in U.S. health care with many insurers and managed-care organizations now offering benefits in this area. Even U.S. medical schools are now offering courses on alternative medicines. Because of consumer demands, physicians are finding that they now need to be educated in this area. In 1990 Americans spent an estimated $14.6 billion on visits to alternative practitioners; in 1997 that amount had increased to $21.2 billion. This survey also estimates that Americans spent $5.1 billion for herbal therapies in 1997. A substantial amount of this money is spent on health promotion or disease prevention rather than on treatment of a specific condition.[1]

Besides the realization that herbal and other alternative therapies are growing, the important information that must be gleaned from these statistics is that the danger exists of drug-herb interactions. It is estimated that less than 40 percent of patients disclose their alternative therapies to their physician. Establishing a good dialogue with your doctor so that potential side effects and interactions can be observed is important. With more usage of herbs and other alternative therapies, better-quality products are made available and more educational opportunities arise for physicians.

Unfortunately, there are many cons in the business of herbal medicine that the consumer must sort through. Because there are no regulations pertaining to selling herbs, as there are for drugs, the marketer of an herb can make just about any claim without having the proof to back it up. This makes it difficult for the consumer. Herbal medicines will never gain the attention of pharmaceutical companies, because they cannot be patented. There is thus no profit to be made from them, at least not to the same degree as for drugs. Would you pay twenty-five dollars for a medicine you could walk out into your backyard and pick? It is doubtful.

Generally speaking, herbal medicine is folk medicine. It is the medicine of the common people—medicine that you and I have access to without involving corporate America or a hierarchy of medical personnel, from nurses and physicians to pharmaceutical companies. People originally put sage in their turkey dressing to prevent botulism and thyme in their pork to kill pinworm; we continue this traditional use today, although we're perhaps no longer aware of the medicinal benefits. In more recent years, people who have used herbal medicines were shunned as too poor or naive to afford a doctor. Now we know that there is a strong scientific basis for herbal medicine.

I know that when I am sick, curling up with a hot cup of herb tea is far more appealing than driving to a doctor's office, sitting for an hour in a waiting room full of other sick people, then climbing onto an examining table to have a cold stethoscope put on my back and chest, only to be given a prescription for antibiotics that probably will not help at all. A healthy lifestyle is all it's cracked up to be. There is no one remedy to compensate for an unhealthy lifestyle. Common sense and moderation must be considered in all things. Your body, too, has inherent mechanisms for maintaining balance; it is called homeostasis. When homeostasis is disrupted, disease occurs.

A SHORT HISTORY OF HERBAL MEDICINE

Human beings have always looked to the plants around them for cures. When the 5,300-year-old mummified Ice Man was found in 1991, his tissues were analyzed. It was found that his rectum was infected with a parasite. Discovered with the Ice Man, tied to a leather thong, were woody fruits of the fungus *Piptoporus betulinus.* This fungus is known to contain antiparasitic properties and was probably used by the Ice Man as a teatment for his rectal parasites.[2] How did people know which plants were therapeutic and which ones were poisonous? Nobody really knows. Surely much of herbal lore was learned through trial and error, and many people became sick from plants. Probably some was learned by watching the animals choose plants. Some healers probably determined plant usage based on intuition or revelations. But plant knowledge for the use of ceremony, magic, and medicine was gained in some way, and passed down verbally through the generations.

Written documents from ancient Egypt, Babylonia, India, and China illustrate medicinal uses of plants. The Chinese emperor Shen Nong, who died in 2697 B.C., made it his responsibility to taste and note the effects of plants on the body to protect his people from poisoning. The early Greeks and Romans wanted to make the use of plants less superstitious and began writing herbals or materia medicas. Herbalists and botanists of that time include Pliny, Theophrastus, Hippocrates, and Dioscorides. Dioscorides, who wrote *De Materia*

Medica in about A.D. 55, was called the "Father of Medical Botany." His text remained the most accurate and most frequently consulted herbal until the sixteenth century, at which time herbals became very popular.

Herbalists of the sixteenth century include John Gerard, John Parkinson, and Nicholas Culpeper. Nicholas Culpeper was criticized for his adherence to the astrological aspects of plants or the Doctrine of Signatures. This system of classification was based on a highly intuitive mode of observation, and thus created many disagreements among professions. Culpeper made a significant contribution, though, in encouraging patients to take responsibility for their own health by using cures that could be found among the plants in their backyards. Although the Doctrine of Signatures may sound a little strange in a modern era of scientific evaluation, much of what was learned through it has proved true. For instance, the root of ginseng strongly resembles a whole human, which suggested its use as a tonic to strengthen all of the body systems. We now have evidence that ginseng has hormonelike effects on the body that are similar to those of steroids.

With the growth of urban culture and the rise of scientific medicine, herbalism again began to get a reputation as being superstitious. It became much easier to synthesize a drug than to find it in nature. The last great herbal was probably *A Modern Herbal* by Maude Grieve, published in 1931. After that, the use of herbs began to decline, and herbal remedies disappeared from pharmacopoeias used by physicians by about 1940. Today there is a great resurgence of interest in herbalism. Part of the resurgence is due to increased interest in our natural world and part is due to acknowledged failures of modern medicine.

IS IT BETTER TO USE HERBS THAN DRUGS?

Although herbs provide many benefits, whether they are better than drugs will probably never be known. There is very little incentive for clinicians to study the efficacy and toxicity of an herbal treatment versus a pharmaceutical drug. Herbs are, however, less expensive. The ethnobotanist Dr. James Duke estimates that for treatment of arthritis, the drug Celebrex costs $2.31 per day, whereas the herbal treatment of curcumin costs 77 cents per day. Echinacea used to treat upper respiratory tract infections costs $1.60 a day, while the new drug Relenza, used for the same symptoms, will cost $42 per day. Herbs also contain a complex array of compounds for treating a given condition, while most pharmaceuticals contain only one isolated compound.

While some people rely solely on the medical establishment to prove the value of any treatment, this is not always the case with widely used drugs. A recent report indicated that clinical trials are often inflated and distorted, resulting in overestimating the efficacy of a drug.[3] This is done by publishing results of the same clinical trial in a number of journals, even though most journals forbid submission of articles that are being published elsewhere. Then, when large meta-analyses are done, the results are distorted. Besides skewing of studies, some treatments become habit, with no studies to back them up, such as the use of antibiotics for treating bronchitis.

Many people are under the impression that any herbal substance is safe. This is absolutely not true. Nature produces potent toxins that kill. Compounds found in plants can also interfere with or add to the effect of prescription drugs. Do not use both herbs and prescription drugs to treat the same disease. The outcome could be worse. It is always best to seek the guidance of an experienced herbalist or health-care practitioner to avoid running into problems with dosages and drug interactions. These topics are beyond the scope of any one book. The hope is that by taking widely available herbs, a problem can be alleviated before powerful prescription drugs become necessary. By using herbs on a regular basis, you become familiar with what they can and cannot do for you. You listen to your body and know what it needs and when.

IS IT BAD TO TAKE ANTIBIOTICS?

Antibiotics have done wonders. Although they have not been responsible for eradicating any specific disease, they have saved lives. Problems arise when they are misused. Today antibiotics are overprescribed for conditions that they will not improve.

A recent survey of practicing physicians confirmed this over-prescribing trend. Prescriptions were analyzed for children presenting with viral conditions that do not benefit from antibiotics. It was found that 44 percent of patients with common colds, 46 percent of patients with upper respiratory tract infections, and 75 percent of patients with bronchitis were prescribed antibiotics.[4] Why is this? An editorial in the *Journal of the American Medical Association* suggests that the reason is a combination of education, experience, expectation, and economics.[5] Many physicians are not aware of the distinguishing symptoms that definitively diagnose bacterial infections and need further education in this area. Family physicians tend to use antibiotics more frequently than do pediatricians because they are less experienced with pediatric patients. This makes them less confident of their diagnostic skills.

Expectations, particularly of parents, often dictate prescription of antibiotics. After taking the time to visit a doctor, many patients or parents of sick children expect, or even demand, to receive a prescription for their efforts. Some physicians admitted that economics, or promoting patient satisfaction and retention, was involved in their decision to prescribe antibiotics. As doctors are expected to see more and more patients with less time to spend with each one, they no longer have much time for discussion of conditions or treatments. Essentially, prescription writing is an efficient use of time. Today, many efforts are under way to educate both physicians and patients on the proper use of antibiotics.

Antibiotic use outside of medicine also affects our health and their ability to remain effective for curing infections. Antibiotics are used in animal husbandry to produce bigger and better animals, even under poor growing conditions, without the inconvenience of disease. The FDA is currently revising its guidelines for the use of antibiotics in animal husbandry to minimize the emergence of bacterial strains that are resistant to antibiotics used in medicine.[6] Although it has long been suspected that the use of antibiotics in animals is directly linked to the occurrence of antibiotic-resistant bacteria in humans, in 1999 there was good proof of that. Quinolone-resistant bacteria, causing diarrhea in humans, were isolated from patients in Minnesota and found to be identical to those bacteria found in chickens that were given quinolone in their feed. Apparently the problem is worse in Europe, as most of these patients had just returned from foreign travel.[7] This is a disturbing discovery.

WHEN SHOULD YOU USE HERBS?

Dr. Merrilee Okey, a D.O. in Colorado, proposes using herbs to treat uncomfortable but not life-threatening diseases. These conditions might include ear and sinus infections as well as bladder and skin infections. Meningitis or bacteremia should never be treated with herbs. Fever, pain, and vomiting are signs of a serious and more immediate disease, says Dr. Okey, and herbs should not be used for these symptoms. Linda B. White, M.D., author of *Kids, Herbs, and Health,* says that disease can take a turn for the worse in children much more quickly than in adults. Be vigilant. If a child less than three months old has a fever, call the doctor immediately. She suggests developing a good relationship with your physician so that you can better discuss when antibiotics are necessary and when they are not.

In Germany, herbalists rarely see patients for infectious disease—they are sent to physicians. Uta Schmidt, an herbalist who practices in Berlin, occasionally treats urinary tract infections and skin infections, such as boils—both of which are self-limiting diseases. When a patient is plagued with chronic infections, she tries to balance their acid-to-base ratio with a special program. It is most important for patients to be responsible for their own bodies, she says, and she tries to help patients see what they can do for themselves.

Linda Millican is an herbalist and the director of Two Moons Herbals in Colorado. She does not claim to be a diagnostician. If you don't know the root of the physical problems you are experiencing, she says, you must see a physician first. Obtaining a diagnosis prevents acute infections from becoming deadly; the correct course of action might be the administration of antibiotics. Millican uses herbs primarily for rebuilding the body rather than for treating trauma. Herbs can help the system function better as well as support the action of drugs. She reminds her patients not to be worried that their allopathic physician does not acknowledge the role that herbs may play in healing, as herbs are not at all a subject of their training. Finally, she asks that patients not be discouraged by the nasty taste of many herbs.

This book explains a number of infectious diseases that could be appropriately treated with herbs. It is advisable, however, to seek medical attention and discuss treatments with a medical doctor. A physician should be on the lookout for worsening of symptoms that require immediate attention.

Do You Need a Physician?

It is often difficult to know when it is appropriate to call a physician or health-care provider. Adults usually know when they are feeling poorly enough, but you don't always know when your child's condition is serious. Children less than a year old can become very sick very fast, and it is better to get an accurate diagnosis from a qualified health

Table 9. Conditions for which to seek immediate medical attention

Disease	Symptoms
Appendicitis	Nausea, vomiting, pain and tenderness in lower-right abdomen, fever
Endocarditis	Pneumonia, fever, increased heart rate, previous infection
Meningitis	Fever, headache, neck and back stiffness, vomiting, confusion, sore throat
Necrotizing fasciitis	Severe pain or loss of feeling at the site of infection, change in skin color, blisters, generalized ill feeling
Septicemia	Current infection that develops into high fever, shaking, chills, weakness, nausea, vomiting, and diarrhea

care provider before any type of treatment is administered. In older children, look for signs of confusion, delirium, loss of consciousness, convulsions, fever of more than 104–106°F, stiffness in the neck, severe pain, signs of dehydration, or inability to swallow. As a parent, you are the one who best knows your child's normal activities; call a doctor if things seem abnormal. After receiving the diagnosis, you can discuss an appropriate treatment. Diseases that can kill quickly, and thus need immediate treatment, include meningitis, necrotizing fasciitis, endocarditis, septicemia, and appendicitis.

APPENDICITIS

Appendicitis can sometimes seem like a bad stomachache, but it requires life-saving surgery. Without surgery, the appendix can burst, sending infectious matter into the abdominal cavity, where it can cause extensive damage. The pain of appendicitis sometimes starts over the stomach and then shifts to the lower-right abdomen. The pain worsens when standing or coughing. Nausea and vomiting are also features of appendicitis. Although appendicitis can be difficult to diagnose, it should be suspected whenever there is severe stomach or abdominal pain.

BACTEREMIA, SEPTICEMIA, AND ENDOCARDITIS

Bacteremia refers to the presence of bacteria in the blood. This can happen simply by clenching the jaw, forcing oral bacteria into the blood. Bacteria can also enter through the intestines. Usually these bacteria are promptly removed by the body's immune system and no symptoms ever develop. But occasionally, bacteria in the blood can lead to an infection that involves many tissues by spreading through the bloodstream. This type of widespread infection is referred to as septicemia, or sepsis. Typically, because of toxins secreted by the bacteria, the entire body is involved in some way. Sepsis can also occur following surgery if sterile procedures were not followed properly, or from the use of catheters in the body. Bacteremia can also lead to endocarditis, or infection of the lining of the heart. Diagnosis of bacterimia is done by drawing blood and analyzing laboratory cultures of that blood. This can take twenty-four to forty-eight hours, which is too long to wait for treatment. As a rule, if septicemia is suspected, antibiotics are started immediately to reduce the chances of death.

MENINGITIS

Meningococcal meningitis is a severe bacterial infection that finds its way to the brain and spinal cord. Although it is rare, outbreaks of the disease do occur. It can spread from person to person by direct contact, sometimes from drinking from the same glass. The most distinguishing characteristic of this disease is a stiff neck that causes severe pain such that it becomes impossible to move the chin to the chest. This is often accompanied by fever, headache, and vomiting. Meningitis can cause permanent damage to the nervous system and sometimes death, if it goes untreated. If meningitis is suspected, cerebrospinal fluid is taken for analysis of the bacteria present.

NECROTIZING FASCIITIS

"Necrotizing" refers to the process of degeneration or death of tissues. The fascia of the body are the membranes that surround individual muscles, giving them support. When these fascia become infected by certain streptococcal bacteria, the result is necrotizing fasciitis. This rapidly spreading and life-threatening disease has been referred to in the press as "flesh-eating strep." Although it is very rare, it demands immediate attention. It causes extreme pain, which may be followed by lack of pain as the nerves are destroyed. The disease is sometimes accompanied by a toxic shock–like syndrome, which affects the respiratory system and may lead to respiratory distress.

PREGNANCY

While it is a normal condition rather than an illness, pregnancy is a delicate time for women, and care should be taken to protect the pregnancy and not to harm the unborn child. For this reason, it is not advisable to ingest caffeine, alcohol, or other drugs. Herbs, too, can have toxic consequences during pregnancy. These herbs, in particular, should not be used during pregnancy: bogbean, borage, burdock, ginseng, goldenseal, juniper, licorice, meadowsweet, myrrh, passionflower, pennyroyal, uva-ursi, and yarrow. Pregnant women should have regular prenatal visits with a trusted health-care provider, be it lay midwife, nurse midwife, physician's assistant, or physician. A medical doctor should be consulted if any warning signs of abnormal pregnancy occur, such as elevated blood pressure, anemia, vaginal bleeding, or sugar detected in the urine. A back-up medical doctor should always be on call during labor and delivery.

6 OTHER MEDICAL TRADITIONS

As Americans, we tend to wait until a disease has reached a point of emergency before seeking medical help. In the past seventy-five years, American medicine, or allopathic medicine, has focused research efforts and funding on emergency types of medicine more than on prevention strategies. Although herbs and folk medicines were once common in practice, they have gradually been replaced by pharmaceutical drugs. Most herbal therapies were discontinued in the United States by the 1940s. The recent renaissance of herbal medicine coincides with revivals in other areas of more holistic medicine as well. Although I have chosen to focus on the immune-strengthening and antibiotic properties of herbal medicine in this book, before discussing specific herbal remedies I would like to give an overview of several other medical traditions and their approaches to infectious disease. These traditions—osteopathic medicine, anthroposophical medicine, hyperthermia, homeopathy, and acupuncture—differ from one another in important ways, but all of them have a more holistic, prevention-oriented focus than does modern Western medicine as it is practiced today. That is, they focus on the whole body as an integrated system, rather than on emergency measures for fighting the specific presenting disease of the moment. And while it is not a medical tradition, I would also like to discuss breast-feeding in this chapter as an important lifelong immune-boosting and disease-preventing strategy.

WHAT IS OSTEOPATHIC MEDICINE?

Osteopathic physicians specialize in manipulative therapy of the musculoskeletal system, especially the head and back. Their training is similar to that of allopathic doctors, or M.D.'s: They first acquire a bachelor's degree and then apply to medical school. Osteopathic medical training is a four-year program in which students study the traditional subjects of anatomy and pathology. The main difference is that they are also trained in manipulation of the bones and muscles, or the musculoskeletal system. On graduation, they are given the degree of doctor of *osteopathy,* or D.O. The word *osteopathy* comes from *osteo,* which means "bone," and *pathos,* which means "suffering or disease." American osteopaths practice in all disciplines of medicine and surgery, with hospital privileges and insurance coverage. Although chiropractors are also trained in manipulation of bones and muscles, their other medical training is far more limited than that of osteopaths.

The field of osteopathy has been with us since 1874, when Andrew T. Still decided to develop a drugless system of therapy based on manipulation. He knew that the body created its own chemicals for healing.[1] We now know that the body does produce many biochemicals, such as prostaglandins and enkephalins, that contribute to both health and disease. Still set up his first school in Kirkersville, Missouri.

Because of Dr. Still's beliefs about drugs, the early osteopathic programs did not teach pharmacology. This was the biggest distinction between them and allopathic medical schools. When allopathic medicine became more popular in the twentieth century, interest in osteopathy declined and the practice responded by becoming more like allopathic medicine. Osteopaths began to learn pharmacology. An important component of osteopathic medicine is treating the body as a connected whole. A physical complaint is not isolated in one part of the body but may be caused by a restriction in another part of the body. Osteopathy addresses movement, such as the movement that occurs within the brain but affects the entire body.

Some osteopaths provide treatment no different from that of allopathic medicine; others focus on using manipulation as a major tool. Osteopathic practitioners believe that the overall structure of the body, meaning the musculoskeletal system, is intimately linked to its function. By addressing issues of the musculoskeletal system, they can heal. A disordered musculoskeletal system can irritate and produce abnormal nerve responses and blood supplies that cause disease in distant organs. By adjusting the mechanical aspects of the body, the circulatory and nervous systems are better able to function, thus removing any restrictions that prevent healing. This method respects the body's natural ability to heal itself. The osteopathic physician strives to treat the patient as a whole rather than just treating his or her symptoms.

When tension and stress settle into the musculoskeletal system, they can waste the body's energy and create a number of health problems. Among the problems that osteopathic medicine is especially skilled at helping are those of the joints, such as arthritis; allergies; chronic cardiac disease; breathing problems; chronic fatigue syndrome; high blood pressure; headaches; and nerve inflammation. During a physical exam, an osteopathic physician will pay particular attention to a patient's posture and motion, the symmetry of the body, and the condition of the muscles and skin. There are several types of manipulation the physician will then use, depending on what is needed. These manipulations include mobilization of a joint slowly through its range of motion; articulation, or a quick thrust of a joint; release methods that allow the patient to relax muscle spasms and other restrictions in the soft tissues; and gentle cranial manipulation of the bones of the head.

Osteopathy is an evolving discipline. One of the most significant contributions was made by William Sutherland in 1939. Realizing that the rhythmic motion of the nervous system is essential for health, he developed craniosacral therapy as a means to modify the primary respiration mechanism.[2] This mechanism describes respiration not only as participated in by the lungs but also on the cellular level. Each cell of the body uses oxygen to make energy in a series of biochemical reactions termed oxidative phosphorylation. Although the head is thought by most people to be immobile, manipulation of the cranial bones, or head bones, affects a number of bodily processes. This adjustment allows for better movement of the cerebral spinal fluid around the brain, thus affecting the spinal column and the twelve pairs of cranial nerves found in the head. This manipulation is a means to release the sacrum, or lower end of the spinal cord, and to balance the head on the spinal cord, which, in turn, allows for better respiration at the cellular level.

The greatest benefits are seen if these manipulations are done shortly after birth, as that is when the body is most responsive. Dr. Viola Frymann, an osteopathic practitioner, says that just the process of birth can cause severe trauma to about 10 percent of newborns. Strains occur in another 78 percent of infants during birth. As a toddler begins walking, the process of falling can cause additional harm by creating strains in the sacrum as well as in the upper vertebrae at the head. Occasional manipulations in children can prevent problems later in life, after the bones are fully formed.[3]

ACUTE INFECTIONS

An osteopathic technique known as the thoracic–lymphatic pump manipulation has been shown to be effective in the treatment of acute bacterial infections. This technique works in a number of ways, including improving lymphatic, arterial, and venous circulations and enhancing lymphatic drainage and leukocyte activity. The physician places his or her hands on the thorax and alternates the pressure applied there. This utilizes the body's natural respiratory movements to increase respiration. This technique was first proved effective in treating patients with the flu during the epidemic of 1918. Human studies have shown that this technique can increase the immune response.[4]

EAR INFECTIONS

Although ear infections are usually treated with antibiotics by most pediatricians, they rarely work and are rarely needed. When otitis media is due to bacterial infection, the infection is present only because of the stagnant fluid that has built up in the ear. According to the osteopathic physician Bob Fulford, fluid in the middle ear stems from restrictions in the sacrum, the lowest vertebra. It is this restriction that prevents the proper flow of lymph, causing fluid to build up in the middle ear. When that fluid stagnates, bacteria grow in it.[5]

Phil Wong, an osteopathic physician practicing in Albuquerque, says that chronic ear infections in children tend to be associated with an imbalance in the temporal bones of the head. This disorder of the bones causes the eustachian tubes, which drain the middle ear, to be misaligned. The chest is also jammed, which decreases the drainage of the lymph from the head and neck. These problems can often be traced back to trauma that occurs during the birthing process, but they can be solved with cranial manipulation. Various other osteopathic manipulations are used to alleviate otitis media. These include soft-tissue releases to facilitate lymphatic drainage around the eustachian tubes, hyoid release, shoulder raising to act as a lymphatic pump, myofacial releases around the mandible, and techniques applied to the cervical vertebrae to improve circulation.[6]

UPPER RESPIRATORY TRACT INFECTIONS

Infections of the upper respiratory tract are characterized by sinusitis, bronchitis, stuffiness in the head, lethargy, fatigue, headaches, and cough. Swelling of the tissues in this area results in decreased circulation, impaired mobility, and altered breathing patterns. Although many physicians are prone to prescribing antibiotics for these conditions, they are futile, as most of these infections are viral in nature. Providing osteopathic manipulation therapy early in the course of disease, however, can shorten the duration of the illness. This normalization of structure can bring about resistance to infection.

Studies conducted by Dr. Ida Schmidt at the Philadelphia College of Osteopathic Medicine have shown that manipulative therapy is useful for treating pharyngitis, rhinitis, and laryngitis. A study conducted on forty-four patients found that osteopathic manipulative therapy was useful for the treatment of pharyngitis, or sore throat. Twenty-five patients treated with manipulative therapy and saltwater gargle were all free of symptoms by the second day. Fourteen patients who were treated with antibiotics and no manipulation took six days to return to health. Another study showed that fifteen patients who were treated with osteopathic manipulative therapy for rhinitis, or runny nose, did not experience further cold symptoms and were still without symptoms the following day.[7]

Some of these manipulations of the face, or myofacial techniques, can be done by patients themselves to increase lymphatic drainage. For pain in the frontal sinuses, lie on your back and rub with your hand back and forth on the forehead just over the eyebrows. Second, using your fingers, make circular motions over the cheekbones, adjacent to the nose. This will be directly over the paranasal sinuses. Also try rubbing just below the eyes, on the cheekbones, and coming up to the bridge of the nose. Last, with one finger, rub down the forehead to the bridge of the nose and, with another finger, rub from the tip of the nose up to the bridge of the nose. These techniques can improve drainage and bring some relief to congested sinuses.

THE FLU EPIDEMIC OF 1918

Osteopathic, or manipulative, therapy was highly successful in treating patients with the flu, also known as the Spanish flu, during the first major epidemic in 1918. Although this was before the advent of antibiotics, these drugs would have done nothing to cure the flu, which is caused by a virus. A survey conducted by the American Osteopathic Association in 1919 found that the mortality rate among osteopathic patients was 0.25 percent, while the mortality rate in the general population was 5 percent, a significant difference. The treatment given to these flu patients was the thoracic–lymphatic pump manipulation. This therapy enhances drainage of the lymph vessels and increases white blood cell activity. In evaluating epidemic-related flu cases that were complicated by pneumonia, osteopathic-treated patients had a mortality rate of 10 percent, compared with 30 percent for allopathic-treated patients. This indicates that osteopathic manipulation also helps in the worse cases of flu, bouts that involve complications.[8]

PNEUMONIA

We have seen that flu patients who experienced pneumonia were successfully treated with osteopathic manipulation. Dr. Wong tells of a patient who came to him after being treated by an allopathic physician for pneumonia. She had already taken two courses of antibiotics and was still suffering neck, chest, and upper-back pain, and the pneumonia and cough associated with it had not improved. After being given osteopathic treatment for the somatic dysfunction in her spine, rib cage, and neck, the respiratory infection subsided within a few days. Dr. Wong says the problem was just due to improper circulation, which prevented the white blood cells as well as the antibiotics from reaching the site of infection.

STRESS

The way the body deals with stress can set it up for infections. Chronic stress weakens the immune system, making it less able to combat an infection. Osteopathic manipulation can bring the nervous system back into alignment during times of stress. By treating the sympathetic nervous system, homeostasis can improve, and the symptoms of stress are minimized. More than just providing relaxation, this manipulation reduces hyperactivity of the sympathetic nerves and allows improved circulation of the blood and lymph. Together, these actions result in a decline in disease and an improvement in health. Reducing this hyperactivity of the sympathetic nervous system by a technique called rib raising can also treat colds and sinus infections.

WHAT IS ANTHROPOSOPHICAL MEDICINE?

This holistic and human-centered approach to medicine was described at the turn of the twentieth century by the German philosopher Rudolf Steiner, who also started the Waldorf school system. It is based on the scientific facts of physiology and bio-chemistry as well as spiritual science and the psyche. This allows for a rational, yet holistic approach to health and disease. While they are M.D.'s, anthroposophical practitioners use many comple-mentary techniques, which include a movement therapy called eurythmy, painting, music, rhythmic massage, and psychological counseling. Most training takes place in Europe, but some regional study groups and teaching situations, or preceptorships, are avail-able in North America.

ANTHROPOSOPHICAL MEDICINE AND
HERBAL MEDICINE

Although most of anthroposophical medicine uses homeopathic rem-edies, herbal remedies are applied as well. The body is roughly di-vided into three parts, each of which is associated with a plant part. The first is the plant root, which tends to be cold and hard; this correlates with the cold, hard sensory and nervous system, which is centered in the head. Next are the leaves of the plant, which are responsible for absorbing and releasing gases. This part is related to the rhythmic system of the body, which is responsible for breathing. Third are the flowers of the plant, which are responsible for repro-duction. This part, in turn, relates to the body's reproductive and metabolic systems.

Rudolf Steiner observed that the plants with the most healing properties also have morphological oddities in their proportions. Medicinal plants seem to have disharmony or imbalance among flower, leaf, and root, much as a diseased person would have among his corresponding parts. For instance, nettles *(Urtica dioica)* have an abundance of leaves, greatly disproportionate to the size of the root system and flowers. It is because of this abundance of foliage that Steiner suggests that the leaves will most affect our rhythmic sys-tem. In fact, nettle is said to strengthen the blood and prevent hemorrhage, thus supporting the rhythmic system of the body. An-other example is chamomile, which produces an abundance of flowers compared with other plant parts. Flowers represent the reproduc-tive aspect of the plant, and this suggests that they would support the reproductive-metabolic system of the body. Chamomile flowers are typically used to calm the digestive tract, which is part of the body's metabolic system.

ANTHROPOSOPHY AND INFECTIOUS DISEASE

The anthroposophical physician Philip Incao believes that health is a balance between the tendency toward inflammation and the tendency toward chronic degenerative disease. Treating or preventing infectious disease is not always necessary, he says; infectious disease and the process of overcoming it can actually benefit a person. With healing, the human soul is enlightened and the spirit is strengthened. In this way, the human spirit evolves and grows stronger. Perhaps this healing from infectious disease prevents the settling in of chronic diseases, such as cancer and asthma, later in life. If you are without disease, the body is not cleaning out its unwanted tissues, which can later cause chronic illnesses. Having a strong immune system fosters inflammation rather than preventing illness. This goes against the standard belief that if you have not been ill for twenty years, you must be healthy. In fact, if you have not been ill for twenty years, believes Dr. Incao, you are probably harboring a chronic disease. The best piece of advice, he says, is to eat good, wholesome foods and practice moderation in life.

A good source of information on anthroposophical medicine is *Spiritual Science and the Art of Healing*, by Victor Bott (*see* "Further Reading").[9]

HYPERTHERMIA

Saunas, hot tubs, or a hot bath may help fight infection by increasing the temperature of the body. This treatment was popularized by Julius Wagner-Jauregg in the early 1900s. To induce fever, Wagner-Jauregg injected malaria into patients, and the ensuing fever was able to cure his patients of syphilis. This won Wagner-Jauregg the Nobel Prize in 1927.[10]

Increasing the body temperature mimics the body's natural process of inducing fever or inflammation. By increasing the temperature, you not only make the environment hostile for infecting microbes but also increase circulation, another health benefit. Rather than inducing malaria, try raising the body temperature by immersing the body in hot water, such as in a bathtub or hot tub; wrapping the body in blankets; or using a sauna or steam bath. Hot baths have a long history of therapeutic use. By increasing the body temperature, you stimulate sweat, which can eliminate toxins that are stored in the body, as well as create a more hostile environment for infectious microbes.[11]

A hot bath can also relieve some of the muscle aches and pains associated with a cold or flu. Enhance the therapeutic value of a bath by adding a few drops of essential oil or a bag of dried herbs. For muscle aches and pains, put a handful of sage and marjoram in a muslin bag under the running hot water. Then use this bag as a washcloth. The therapeutic compounds in the herbs will be dispersed in the tub and help relieve symptoms. Remember to drink plenty of cool water after you get out of the bath, and keep yourself warm for a few minutes. Care should be taken to keep the body temperature below 102°F. This treatment should not be undertaken by those with a heart condition, pregnant women, or diabetics. A low-temperature sauna, 105–110°F, will have the same effect. Some people have seen good results from staying in a sauna for thirty to forty-five minutes a day for several weeks.

HOMEOPATHY

Homeopathy, begun in the late eighteenth century by the German physician Samuel Hahnemann, is based on the principle of similars; that is, a highly diluted dose of a substance that causes your disease or condition can actually cure the disease. In the case of infection, a highly diluted bacterium might be administered. For instance, to treat the itching associated with chicken pox, a dilution from the poison ivy plant might be used. Homeopathic treatment uses very toxic substances, such as heavy metals, but, in theory, the concentration of these substances is negligible.

In addition, homeopathy calls for treating each patient in a unique way, based on the individual's constitution. For this reason, homeopathy cannot be self-prescribed, as the constitution of an individual must be determined by a skilled homeopathic practitioner. Reviews of the effectiveness of homeopathic medicine have repeatedly been performed, and the results are consistently inconclusive. Nonetheless, many people have found homeopathy beneficial. A popular homeopathic treatment for symptoms of the flu is oscillococcinum. It acts to stimulate the body's own defenses to relieve the discomforts of flu. This remedy is widely used in France.

ACUPUNCTURE

Acupuncture therapy has received a lot of interest in the United States recently, with more than one million Americans receiving this treatment each year. The National Institutes of Health (NIH) in 1997 reviewed the literature regarding acupuncture and concluded that although there were some difficulties interpreting data due to the lack of appropriate controls, acupuncture is effective in relieving the pain associated with many conditions, such as arthritis. It recommends more research to determine other appropriate areas for acupuncture therapy. The NIH is now funding several research programs employing acupuncture, including one using acupuncture for the treatment of respiratory diseases, including bronchitis.

Acupuncture is an ancient Chinese therapy that is typically used to alleviate pain, but it is also used to increase immunity. The theory of acupuncture is based on the presence of energy channels, also called meridians, that flow through the body. When the flow of energy in any given meridian becomes disrupted, disease can occur. Acupuncture stimulates specific locations on the skin, usually with needles but also with electrical impulses, smoke, pressure, heat, or lasers. Research has shown that stimulating these points causes specific biological reactions mediated by sensory neurons within the central nervous system. For instance, neurotransmitters and neurohormones are released. The hypothalamus and pituitary gland are also activated. Changes in blood flow and alterations in immune function have also been seen.[12]

The NIH concluded that the data in support of acupuncture were just as strong as for many of the well-accepted Western medical therapies. But one important advantage of acupuncture is that the incidence of side effects is much lower than it is in many drugs or other procedures used to treat the same conditions. The World Health Organization recognizes the use of acupuncture for several infectious diseases, including diarrhea, respiratory illness, colds, tonsillitis, sinusitis, sore throat, bronchitis, and lung infections. Besides the institutes that train laypeople in acupuncture, there are now many opportunities for allopathic M.D.'s to be taught in the art of acupuncture and to use it as part of their practice. Some insurance companies, as well, are beginning to accept acupuncture and cover its costs.

To perform acupuncture, the practitioner inserts small needles through the skin into the acupuncture points on the body, where they usually remain for twenty to thirty minutes. The number of treatments a patient requires depends on the person and the illness being treated. Acupuncture is now being used to treat chronic diseases including AIDS. There is evidence that acupuncture can have a beneficial effect on the immune system and on treating infectious disease as well.[13, 14] Accupuncture can also be done in combination with other treatments to improve their efficacy or to decrease side effects.

Although acupuncture requires a trained professional and is not something you can do yourself, there is a practice similar to acupuncture, called acupressure or shiatsu. Acupressure involves applying deep pressure to the meridians rather than needles. Bodywork of this type can also stimulate the flow of lymph and improve circulation. A qualified practitioner can teach individuals how to perform some types of acupressure on themselves.

BREAST-FEEDING

Breast-feeding can be the best gift you give to your children, with benefits lasting their entire lives. Breast-feeding has been scientifically shown to reduce the risk of many illnesses in children, including diarrhea; respiratory tract, ear, blood, and urinary tract infections; and enterocolitis. A newborn also gains immunological benefits from the transfer of immunoglobulins and white blood cells from its mother. In fact, an infant does not effectively make his or her own immunoglobulins until about the age of six months; until that time, the mother's breast milk is a major source of protection. The normal flora in the intestines of breast-fed babies is also more protective than that of babies fed cow's milk. Breast-feeding may also improve mental development and thus the overall intelligence of a child. Allergies also are minimized in the breast-fed baby. The benefits to child, mother, and even the environment (no packaging to dispose of) are limitless and cannot be discussed at length here.

The American Academy of Pediatrics suggests breast-feeding infants for a full twelve months; this provides benefits to mothers, infants, families, and society. Scientific evidence supports that there are health, nutritional, immunological, developmental, psychological, social, economic, and environmental advantages to breast-feeding. The academy warns, though, that mothers with active and untreated tuberculosis, those who use illegal drugs, and those with HIV infections should not breast-feed. These dangers, however, are not well established. Also, mothers taking certain prescription drugs may want to temporarily stop breast-feeding.[15]

HERBS THAT PROMOTE MILK PRODUCTION

If you have made the decision not to breast-feed based on fears of inadequate milk supply, there are herbs that can help you. Successful breast-feeding also depends on getting enough rest and relaxation. Try drinking a cup of soothing herb tea to help you relax when breast-feeding—perhaps one containing chamomile. An occasional beer with a high hops content may also help you relax. Make an herb pillow filled with hops, chamomile, and lavender to put inside your pillowcase to promote rest and sleep. Try a bath or massage using essential oils to promote relaxation—lavender oil is a good choice. Together, these suggestions may help you enjoy breast-feeding.

Some herbs that promote milk production are:

Aniseed *(Pimpinella anisum)*
Fennel *(Foeniculum vulgare)*
Fenugreek *(Trigonella foenum-graecum)*

Follow the guidelines below to ensure a successful breast-feeding experience.

- Begin as soon as possible after giving birth.
- Nurse whenever the infant appears to want to nurse, eight to twelve times every twenty-four hours.
- Do not give the baby any supplements, such as water, juice, or formula.
- Avoid pacifiers to prevent nipple confusion.
- Air-dry your nipples to prevent cracking and infection.
- Eat nourishing food, be sure to drink plenty of liquids.
- Get enough rest.

7 HERBAL TREATMENT OF SPECIFIC CONDITIONS

ACNE

Acne has been the bane of many teenagers, affecting their social lives and self-esteem. Most people suffer from acne at some time in their lives, but usually during adolescence. Acne, an inflammation of the sebaceous, or oil, glands of the skin, occurs primarily on the face but also on the shoulders, upper chest, and back. We don't know exactly what causes it, but it can be activated by the hormones produced during puberty. The same hormones that are responsible for spurring overall body growth also stimulate the growth of oil glands. This increased oil production blocks the pores and creates an environment conducive to bacterial growth. The bacterium responsible is *Propionibacterium acnes,* a gram-positive organism.

Mild acne takes the form of small, pus-filled pustules called whiteheads. Sometimes the sebum in the glands turns black when exposed to air, creating what is referred to as a blackhead. More severe acne appears as swellings, or nodules. A nodule appears when the pore of the oil gland closes and inflammation occurs inside the gland.

Acne can also form cysts, which cause scarring. Although this condition is usually outgrown, it can be demoralizing because of the effect it has on the appearance.

Acne is often treated with long-term topical and oral antibiotics. Oral antibiotics include tetracycline, erythromycin, and minocycline. Long-term use of tetracycline and erythromycin has been associated with failure of oral contraceptives—an effect that sexually active acne sufferers must bear in mind. These antibiotics are also not appropriate to take during pregnancy. Long-term use of antibiotics can severely alter the normal flora throughout the body and cause yeast infections and gastric disturbances.

Usually, acne goes away even if left untreated, but there are ways to lessen its severity other than with antibiotics. Because increased oil production seems to be at the heart of bacterial growth, keeping the face clean and free of excess oil is important. Remember that using an alkaline soap removes the natural protective acid layer of the skin; this acid pH should be restored with a toner. (Recipes for vinegar-based toners can be found in chapter 9). Although the role of diet in the development of acne is not well established, it is probably wise to pay attention to any connection you might find between food and acne flare-ups. If you notice that eating a certain food is followed by a worsening of acne, cut that food out of the diet. Pay particular attention to chocolate, refined sugars, fried foods, and margarine. Try adding foods or supplements to your diet that contain vitamin A, zinc, vitamin E, selenium, vitamin B_6, vitamin C, and pantothenic acid (*see* table 10).

TREATING ACNE WITH ESSENTIAL OILS

Acne can be treated topically in a number of ways. Tea tree oil has significant antiseptic and disinfectant properties (*see* monograph in chapter 8). A single-blind, randomized study on 124 patients showed that 5 percent tea tree oil in water was nearly as effective as 5 percent benzoyl peroxide, but without the negative side effects.[1] Those with more severe acne can use a more concentrated solution, 10 percent or more. Tea tree oil is one of the few essential

Table 10. Food Sources for Nutrients

Nutrient	Food Source
Vitamin A	Dandelion greens, lamb's-quarter, kale, carrots, broccoli, collard greens, pumpkin, sorrel or dock, sweet potato, apricots
Vitamin B	Whole grains and beans (legumes), brewer's yeast
Vitamin C	Peas, oranges, broccoli, parsley, strawberries
Vitamin E	Wheat germ oil, walnut oil, sunflower oil, safflower oil, almonds, spinach, sweet potato, wild blackberries
Manganese	Tea *(Camellia sinensis)*, nuts, wheat germ, leafy green vegetables
Pantothenic acid	Whole grains, beans, broccoli, brewer's yeast
Selenium	Wheat germ, Brazil nuts, whole grains
Zinc	Legumes, whole grains, shellfish

oils that are safe to apply full strength to the skin. Because many of the essential oils have strong antibacterial properties, others may also prove effective; however, no clinical studies have investigated the effect of other oils on acne. Oils that may have a more acceptable smell and be easier to use include bergamot, chamomile, lavender, thyme, rosemary, and myrrh. Except for lavender, these oils also need to be diluted to a 5 percent solution. Add fifteen drops of oil to about a tablespoon of water and wipe the face with a soaked cotton ball.

A Personal Account

After struggling with acne for several years, and with the side effects of many of the treatments, Lauren decided to draw the line when her physician suggested antibiotics. Rather, she decided to try herbal remedies. She began washing her face twice daily with diluted cider vinegar infused with yarrow flowers. At night she dabbed straight tea tree oil directly onto each pimple and applied rose clay on top of that to help it dry out. Within a few days, her acne had cleared up. Now she continues to maintain her complexion with the daily washings with diluted infused vinegar and only occasionally needs to use the tea tree oil and clay.

USEFUL HERBS TO USE ON OILY SKIN

Several herbs have a drying affect and can reduce the amount of excess oil on the skin. Make a strong herbal tea to apply to your face after cleansing. Alternatively, extract any of these herbs in vinegar for a toner to use after cleansing. Herbs that are useful for treating oily skin include:

Clary sage *(Salvia scarea)*
Lavender (*Lavendula* spp.)
Lemon balm *(Melissa officinalis)*
Red clover *(Trifolium pratense)*
Rosemary *(Rosmarinus officinalis)*
Sage *(Salvia officinalis)*
Strawberry leaves (*Fragaria* spp.)
Tansy *(Tanacetum vulgare)*
Yarrow *(Achillea millefolium)*

ATHLETE'S FOOT AND
FUNGAL SKIN INFECTIONS

The burning, itching feeling of athlete's foot is quite common. Athlete's foot is one of a group of skin diseases also called tinea or ringworm, owing to the appearance of the accompanying skin lesions. These lesions appear as a round, scaly area of skin, with an enlarged outer margin and a clear inner area. Depending on their location on the body, each has a different name. Tinea capitis is a scalp infection often found in schoolchildren. Tinea cruris is an infection of the genital area, also referred to as jock itch. Tinea barbae affects the area of the beard. Tinea unguium or onychomycosis is an infection of the toenail or fingernail. Because of the slow growth of nails, these infections are usually very resistant to treatment. Tinea pedis is classic athlete's foot.

All of these skin infections are caused by various fungi belonging to the genera *Microsporum, Trichophyton,* and *Epidermophyton.* Each gives rise to very superficial skin disease, infecting only the outer layer of skin. Athlete's foot affects the feet, especially the area between the toes. It can produce itching, redness, and vesicles on the skin that rupture. With time, there is scaling, thickening of the skin, and cracking. The risk of bacterial infection increases with the appearance of cracks. Although anyone can get these dermatophytic infections, they are more prevalent in warm, humid climates and in men between the ages of twenty and forty.[2]

More serious fungal infections affect the lower layers of skin, sometimes invading the blood and spreading to other organs. If you have open skin lesions, fever, or raised bumps on the skin, or if an infection does not clear up with treatment, see a physician. Fungal diseases can be deadly. They should clear up within two to three weeks, though infections of the hands and feet can take longer to heal. Mainstream treatments for skin disease include topical antifungal agents, such as ketoconazole, ciclopirox, naftifine, and tolnaftate. These drugs may irritate the skin, leading to stinging, itching, redness, drying of the skin, and allergic reactions.[3]

One way to lower the risk of these fungal, or dermatophytic, infections is to keep the skin dry. Fungus grows best in warm, moist areas. Because these fungal infections usually affect just the outer layer of skin, it is best to use a topical rather than an oral treatment. By applying a remedy directly to the infection, you decrease the risk of side effects. Herbal topical treatments include goldenseal, chamomile, tea tree oil, and garlic. Echinacea, taken orally, can also help clear up a fungal infection.

GOLDENSEAL

Goldenseal *(Hydrastis canadensis)* has a long history of use against fungal infections. Its antimicrobial activity is due its potent alkaloids, primarily hydrastine and berberine. Goldenseal is best used topically, as it works best when in direct contact with the pathogen. Apply goldenseal as a poultice dusted directly onto the skin. Although few scientific studies have been undertaken to validate the effectiveness of goldenseal against fungal infections, berberine has been shown to be effective against many fungal species.[4] Another herb that contains berberine is bloodroot *(Sanguinaria canadensis)*. This herb has demonstrated effectiveness against skin fungi and is an anti-inflammatory agent as well. Additional herbs[5] that may be useful against fungal infections because of their berberine content include Oregon grape *(Berberis aquifolium)*, shrub yellow root *(Xanthorrhiza simplicissima)*, barberry *(Berberis vulgaris)*, and goldthread *(Coptis chinensis, C. groenlandica)*.[6]

CHAMOMILE

A component of the essential oil of German chamomile *(Matricaria recutita)*, chamazulene, has both antiseptic and anti-inflammatory properties.[7] The anti-inflammatory activity stems from its ability to inhibit the production of inflammatory prostaglandins.[8] The essential oil of chamomile can be applied directly to the skin or diluted in oil, water, or cream. A chamomile cream (Kamillosan) was shown to be effective in relieving inflammation associated with dermatosis.[9] Chamomile can be found in many skin creams and is good for prevention of skin infections, particularly in light of its lack of toxic effects. Apply it when the skin becomes cracked from itching.

TEA TREE OIL

Tea tree oil is the essential oil from various species of *Melaleuca*. It has been found to be active against most forms of fungus that cause skin infections.[10, 11] In a double-blind, randomized trial that included 104 patients with athlete's foot, a 10 percent tea tree oil solution relieved the symptoms of athlete's foot as well as did the antifungal medication tolnafate.[12] Another double-blind, randomized clinical trial compared the effectiveness of tea tree oil to a popular prescription treatment for toenail fungus, clotrimazole. The results showed that tea tree oil was an effective, safe, and inexpensive treatment for toenail fungus, or onchomycosis.[13] It can be applied full strength to the toenail, but should be diluted for skin applications. Never take tea tree oil internally.

GARLIC

Garlic *(Allium sativum)* has a history of use in the treatment of ring-worm, and scientific evidence backs up this application. An aqueous extract of garlic was found to be effective against 90 percent of the organisms that cause tinea infections.[14] One study found that the purified component, ajoene, inhibited the growth of a wide range of fungi.[15] Another study evaluating the effect of a cream containing 0.4 percent ajoene showed that 79 percent of patients with athlete's foot were free of fungus after just seven days of treatment.[16]

CLOVE

Clove *(Syzygium aromaticum)* has many antimicrobial properties. A tincture of cloves made in 70 percent alcohol has been successful in treating athelete's foot.[17]

ECHINACEA

Echinacea *(Echinacea angustifolia, E. pallida,* or *E. purpurea)* is one of the most widely used herbs. It stimulates the immune response, which can support the body in fighting any chronic infection, such as athlete's foot. It is usually recommended that echinacea extract be taken three times a day during an active infection.[18]

OTHER REMEDIES

Sage, rosemary, and thyme also have a history of use as antifungal agents, and their effectiveness has been confirmed in laboratory studies but not in human trials.[19]

BODY ODOR

With the exception of bad breath (*see* gingivitis section in this chapter), body odor usually originates from the skin. The body produces two types of sweat from two types of sweat glands—eccrine sweat glands and apocrine sweat glands. Most body odor is a result of bacteria that thrive on secretions from the apocrine sweat glands. These glands begin to function at puberty. They are located primarily under the arms and in the pubic area. Rather than reacting just to heat, these glands react to stress, anger, nervousness, and sexual excitement, even producing a "cold sweat." When sweat is excreted from these glands, skin bacteria grow and multiply, digesting this sweat as well as the dead layer of skin. This decomposition is what produces the odor of sweat. The best way to eliminate odor is with good hygiene. Sometimes, however, a good daily washing is simply not enough, so we resort to other measures.

Many people today use deodorants and antiperspirants. These agents usually contain metals that, when absorbed into the body, can be somewhat toxic and may cause skin irritation. Antibacterial herbs can also be used. An easy way to use herbs for body odor is to combine them with body powder. Both sage and rosemary have antibacterial properties[20] and a rather nice smell themselves. Mix a few teaspoonfuls of ground herb with a cup of a mixture of half cornstarch and half baking soda (*see* chapter 9). Apply this mixture to your body after showering to minimize body odors.

Other causes of body odor include general poor health and gastrointestinal problems. More specifically, a particular bacterium in the stomach called *Helicobacter* can be responsible for some cases of gastritis and ulcers. If the body odor is ammonia-like, it could be caused by this form of bacteria. Treatment for *Helicobacter* is discussed in this chapter in the section on ulcers. Body odor can also be the result of skin infections. The most common is athlete's foot. If your feet smell, consider one of the treatments discussed in this chapter in the section on athlete's foot.

Other conditions that may cause body odor include metabolic problems that arise from eating too much protein or too much fat. To eliminate these odors, it is important to eat whole foods, less protein, and less fat. Ingesting probiotics, such as yogurt, might restore health to the digestive tract and minimize odors that originate from the mouth. Eating fennel after a meal can improve digestion and alleviate bad breath caused by poor digestion. This remedy was suggested as early as the twelfth century by the German mystic Hildegard von Bingen. A short-term herbal detoxification program can be recommended by an herbalist to help eliminate body odors as well.

BRONCHITIS

Constant coughing that brings up sputum is a sign of bronchitis, an inflammation of the bronchial tubes, which enter the lung. Even though 95 percent of cases of acute bronchitis are caused by viruses, a recent survey showed that antibiotics are the most common treatment.[21, 22] Bronchitis typically lasts seven to ten days, but it may last more than a month. Bronchitis that holds on for three months or longer is considered chronic bronchitis. Bronchitis can also result from asthma, chemical irritants, or bacterial infection. When bronchitis is due to a bacterial infection, *Mycoplasma pneumoniae* is usually the causative agent of acute bronchitis; *Streptococcus pneumonia, Haemophilus influenzae,* and *Moraxella catarrhalis* are the leading pathogens found with chronic bronchitis.[23] The most significant risk factor for chronic bronchitis, however, is cigarette smoking.

Using antibiotics such as erythromycin, doxycycline, trimethoprim, and sulfamethoxazole to treat bronchitis is the subject of controversy in the medical community. Many studies show that antibiotics do not improve acute or chronic bronchitis, even when bronchitis is caused by *Mycoplasma pneumoniae.*[24] The evidence in favor of antibiotics is somewhat stronger in cases of chronic bronchitis, however. Patients with this condition are more susceptible to bacterial infection because of continual irritation of the airways. This can progress to infection of the lung by pneumonia. The mortality rate with pneumonia was 30 percent before the advent of antibiotics.[25] In many cases, the reason for administering antibiotics is that the patient expects to receive them. In others, the physician prescribes them prophylactically, as a way to prevent a bacterial infection. This widespread use of antibiotics has led to the emergence of penicillin-resistant *Streptococcus pneumoniae,* which is now more difficult to treat.[26] This is a particular concern because this same organism can cause meningitis and ear infections in children. Bacteria that can give rise to chronic bronchitis are *S. pneumoniae, Haemophilus influenzae,* and *Moraxella catarrhalis.* Bear in mind that bacterial causes are found in only 50 percent of patients with chronic bronchitis. Other drugs besides antibiotics are widely used to treat bronchitis as well. These include bronchodilators to increase airflow to the lungs and steroids to decrease inflammation.

An important part of treating chronic bronchitis is to open the airways that have become blocked by inflammation. First, any irritants, such as tobacco smoke, chemicals, and allergens in the home, must be removed. Airways can be blocked by excessive mucus. Improve your nutrition (dairy products tend to be mucus forming for many people), and drink plenty of water. The respiratory muscles also need to be strengthened by gradually developing an exercise program. Walking may be the best way to start. Often, theophylline is prescribed to help dilate or expand the airways. This drug is also found in black tea and in orange pekoe tea.

Another goal of treatment is to expel the mucous secretions from the lungs, an objective that is defeated when cough suppressants are used. Agents that work to expel mucus are called expectorants. Their job is threefold: to increase the quantity of, decrease the viscosity of, and promote the expulsion of secretions from the lungs. Use herbs that act as expectorants. The most common example is probably eucalyptus. It not only has expectorant properties, but also is an antibacterial and antiviral agent.[27] Once smoked as a treatment for respiratory problems, the essential oil is now used in diffusers and steam. Put a few drops of eucalyptus oil in a pan of hot water. Place your head over the pan and breath in the vapors. Besides acting as an expectorant, eucalyptus has antiseptic properties and can dilate the bronchioles. Do not take the oil internally, however; it can be toxic. Eucalyptus can also be diluted in oil or ointment and rubbed on the chest to promote clearing of mucus (*see* chapter 9 for a decongestant salve recipe).

Elecampane *(Inula helenium)* was once listed in the U.S. Pharmacopoeia as a treatment for afflictions of the respiratory organs.[28] It is known to relax the tracheal smooth muscle, which allows more airflow to the lungs.[29] Its antibacterial properties have also been documented.[30] It is typically used as a liquid extract of the root or rhizome.

Horehound *(Marrubium vulgare)* also has a history of use for bronchitis and sore throats. It promotes expulsion of phlegm and can quiet a cough as well.[31] Although horehound grows as a weed in many areas, it can make a nice addition to your medicinal herb garden. It is also easily available in cough drops.

Yerba Santa *(Eriodictyon californicum),* the Holy Herb, has a tradition of use for the treatment of chronic bronchitis, colds, and asthma.[32]

Licorice *(Glycyrrhiza glabra)* has traditionally been used to treat bronchitis and respiratory infections. It also acts as an expectorant, helping bring up mucus from the lungs.[33] Licorice is available in many forms—as a candy, tea, tincture, and powder. You can also suck on a piece of root. Take care not to overuse licorice, however; too much may cause water retention and increased blood pressure. The safer form of licorice mentioned earlier, known as deglycyrrhizinated licorice, is not effective for treating bronchitis. On the other hand, it can be used for conditions of the digestive tract.

Plantain *(Plantago major)* is useful for treating bronchitis as well. Ironically, the plants we consider to be weeds and most often try to rid from our yards frequently end up being the most beneficial. Plantain is one of those. Although usually thought of as a laxative and cholesterol-lowering agent, plantain has a history of use in treating chronic bronchitis. It can dilate the bronchi, allowing more air to reach the lungs; it can inhibit inflammation; and it has antibacterial properties.[34] A recent study indicates that extracts from plantain can inhibit prostaglandin synthesis. Prostaglandins are fatty acids involved in inflammation. An older study, published in Bulgaria,

TABLE 11. EXPECTORANT HERBS

Herb	Preparation
Elecampane *(Inula helenium):*	Drink a sip at a time of a decoction made from the root.
Eucalyptus *(Eucalyptus globulus):*	Inhale the vapors of the essential oil.
Horehound *(Marrubium vulgare):*	Drink as a cold tea, one cup per day by the spoonful.
Licorice *(Glycyrrhiza glabra):*	Drink a sip at a time of a decoction made from the root or chew on the root.
Lobelia *(Lobelia inflata):*	Use as a tincture. The U.S. FDA warns that this herb contains toxic alkaloids.
Plantain *(Plantago major):*	Drink one to three cups of tea made from the leaves daily, or use as a tincture.
Thyme *(Thymus vulgaris):*	Drink as a tea with honey three times a day. Honey will also provide benefits due to its soothing and antibacterial properties.[41]
Yerba Santa *(Eriodictyon californicum):*	Drink a sip at a time as a strong tea made from the leaves.

showed that plantain was effective in relieving symptoms[35] of chronic bronchitis with no toxic effects.[36]

Thyme *(Thymus vulgaris)* has properties as an antitussive and expectorant and has been used as a treatment for bronchitis.[37] Oil from thyme has proven antibacterial activity.[38] Thyme can be used as a tea; its essential oil can be used in a diffuser.

Garlic *(Allium sativum)* has many antimicrobial properties as well as immunostimulant activity. It is a traditional treatment for bronchitis. Because its active agents and volatile oils are secreted through the lungs after ingestion, garlic may be an effective treatment for upper respiratory tract infections when eaten.[39]

Angelica *(Angelica archangelica)* is another herb with a history of use for treating bronchitis. It has both anti-inflammatory and antibacterial properties.[40]

When bronchitis is a secondary result of asthma, complications can include infection of the airways. Asthma can be triggered by a number of things, including allergens. Try to keep your home free of allergens. The most common household allergens are the dust mites found in carpets and pillows. Asthma patients need to pay particular attention to preventing infections of the airway because they are quite susceptible to such allergens. Signs of more severe lung disease include coughing up blood or bloody mucus and wheezing that persists for a week or more. If you have these symptoms, see a physician. Chemical irritants can trigger asthma as well. Common chemical irritants include:

- Aerosol sprays, such as hairspray and deodorant
- Air pollution with high levels of sulfur dioxide
- Dusts
- Gases in the workplace

COLD SORES/HERPES

Cold sores, sometimes called fever blisters, are lesions that are usually found in or near the mouth and nose. They are caused by a virus called herpes simplex virus 1 (HSV-1). The growth of HSV-1, and subsequently of cold sores, is triggered by ultraviolet light, hormonal changes, and emotional stress. This virus is related to herpes simplex virus 2 (HSV-2), which is responsible for lesions in the genital area. Patients can be infected with either type of herpes and not show symptoms but still be able to transmit the disease. The skin lesions associated with herpes are groups of small, usually painful vesicles. These lesions become crusted after about a week.

Herpes infections are transmitted only by direct contact with the broken skin or mucous membranes of someone who is infected. To prevent herpes, eliminate contact with anyone who has open sores.

Keep your skin in good shape to limit the ability of the virus to penetrate it. Once you are infected with herpes, it can remain dormant and then flare up and cause lesions at any time.

The antiviral medication acyclovir is a nucleoside analog and works by inhibiting replication of the virus. Acyclovir is increasingly being prescribed for cold sores, so much so that the medical community is concerned about resistant herpesviruses. There have been several different mutations identified as acyclovir-resistant herpes. Although this might not sound too serious, given the relatively self-limited course of a cold sore, herpesviruses can also cause infections of the eye that may result in blindness. Herpes can also precipitate encephalitis, which could lead to death. The side effects of acyclovir are not negligible either; they include neurological and kidney toxicities.[42] There are two useful herbs that you can subsitute: melissa and cloves.

Melissa, or lemon balm *(Melissa officinalis)*, has shown activity against herpesvirus[43] and clinical studies on lemon balm and herpes undertaken in Germany have reported positive results as well.[44] See the recipe in chapter 9 for a lip balm made with melissa, or use a commercial lip balm preparation that contains melissa extracts. Apply this lip balm regularly to prevent cold sores, or use it when an outbreak occurs to decrease the extent of the sores.

Cloves *(Syzygium aromaticum)* also have been found to have anti-herpes effects in laboratory studies. When given orally, extracts of clove were able to inhibit the formation of herpes (HSV-1) lesions in mice. A compound in cloves called eugeniin exhibits antiviral activity toward four different strains of HSV-1, the virus that causes cold sores.[45] It works differently from acyclovir in that it inhibits viral DNA synthesis. Cloves contain pain-relieving ingredients useful against cold sores as well.[46] When you feel the first itch of a cold sore, put a clove bud between your lips and keep it there as much as possible for a day or so, until the symptoms have passed. This can prevent the cold sore from becoming established.

A component of licorice root *(Glycyrrhiza glabra)*, glycyrrhetinic acid, is often recommended by herbalists as a topical treatment for herpes. This compound has antiviral activity against a variety of viruses, including HSV-1.[47] Commercial glycyrrhetinic acid creams are available. Make sure you do not use a deglycyrrhizinated licorice product for cold sores, however; it will be missing the important ingredient. You can also try holding a piece of licorice root between your lip and gum.

Echinacea also has anti-herpes activity. It can be used topically directly on a lesion as well as orally to stimulate the immune system. A commercial cream (Viracea) combines echinacea extract with benzaldonium chloride as a treatment for herpes 1 and 2.[48]

Sandalwood *(Santalum album)* essential oil has activity against both HSV-1 and HSV-2.[49] If you prefer, incorporate this oil into a lip balm.

Other nutritionally based treatments include supplementing your diet with zinc, vitamin B, and vitamin C during the outbreak of a cold sore.

COMMON COLD

While it is a relatively benign infection, a cold can make you feel miserable for several days. The common cold is caused by a number of viruses that infect the nose, including rhinoviruses and adenoviruses. It is more correctly called viral rhinitis. Because of the almost infinite number of subtypes of these viruses, people remain susceptible to colds throughout life. This susceptibility is in contrast to the other viruses, such as measles, where immunity can be achieved after an initial infection. Most people feel the effects of a cold once or twice a year. The first symptoms of a cold are similar to those of a number of diseases; they include headache, nasal congestion, watery eyes and nose, sneezing, and scratchy throat. Colds are usually accompanied by a feeling of exhaustion or at least tiredness. A few complications can arise from a cold, including fluid in the middle ear and bacterial infection, and care should be taken to prevent these.

So far neither conventional nor alternative medicine has been able to produce a cure for the common cold. This is not to say that cold treatments are not available; in fact, everyone seems to have his or her own favorite. Mine is just old-fashioned rest! It seems that when I have a cold, my body is telling me to slow down and take a break. Although this is sometimes difficult to do in a world in which we seem to have so many commitments, a cold is the time to pick your least favorite chore and give it up for a nap. Many cold treatments are similar to those for bronchitis, as symptoms are similar, so be sure to read that section as well.

Take note if you use over-the-counter nasal sprays that contain oxymetazolone (Afrin) or phenylephrine (Allerest). Although these sprays provide almost immediate relief from nasal congestion, they are also somewhat addictive. After a few days of use they can lead to more severe congestion that becomes chronic. Side effects can also include headache, excitability, and restlessness.[50]

Echinacea *(Echinacea purpurea* or *E. angustifolia)* is commonly used for preventing colds. It has been shown to be effective in activating immune cells in culture and a few clinical studies have shown that echinacea can reduce the duration and severity of colds.[51] Research has not determined the best way to use exhinacea or how much echinacea works best. Until more specific information becomes available, the recommended dosage is 2–3 milliliters of expressed juice, two to three times a day, at the first sign of a cold.

Many herbs can be drunk as a tea to provide relief. While drinking, inhale the warm vapors into the nasal passages and lungs. This will help moisten and soothe the tissues. Mint may help alleviate some symptoms of a cold, as it can reduce the amount of mucus.[52] Use any species of mint—peppermint and catnip are particularly recommended. Catnip is a popular herb to promote sweating, which can help a cold.[53] Elecampane *(Inula helenium)* also promotes sweating and has been used for colds. It is also good for a cough and has antibacterial properties.[54] The root of elecampane is used in tea or it can be taken as a liquid extract. A favorite of many is a brew made from the gingerroot *(Zingiber officinale)*, which warms the body, relieves pain, and soothes the stomach.[55] Add maple syrup and it makes a delicious tea.

Herbs for colds can also be taken in foods. Often the taste buds become deadened with a cold, and the extra spice can help you enjoy your food. Garlic stimulates the immune system and has antibacterial and antiviral effects.[56] Use garlic heavily in foods while you have a

A Personal Account

Marty is a tax accountant. He knows that every April will bring stress and weaken his immune system, leaving him more vulnerable to disease. After repeating this cycle of stress followed by days off for colds, he has learned how to keep himself healthy. In March, Marty begins strengthening his immune system by first cutting back on sugar and including more whole grains in his diet. He makes a root-vegetable stew that includes slices of immune-stimulating astragalus root, several cloves of garlic, and an onion, which he eats at least once a week. In addition, he increases his vitamin C intake with 500 milligram vitamin C supplements and by drinking tea rich in vitamin C each day. This tea includes rose hips, orange peel, and dandelion leaves, and is sweetened with honey. If the slightest sign of a cold appears, Marty keeps it at bay with echinacea and zinc. He also tries to incorporate more exercise into his schedule. One way he does this is by parking two blocks from the office, then walking briskly from his car to work. This also gives him time to clear his thoughts. Since integrating these practices, Marty hasn't become ill in April or May.

cold. Turmeric *(Curcuma longa)* can relieve cold symptoms as well as aches and pains.[57] Cayenne pepper *(Capsicum frutescens)* has the ability to reduce nasal congestion and relieve pain.[58] All three of these herbs are used liberally in East Indian cooking. A cold treatment used by the Native Americans of the southwestern United States and Mexico is osha *(Ligusticum porteri)*, also known as Porter's lovage. Sniffing the root is said to clear congestion in the nose, and a tea made from the root can cure colds and fever.[59] Osha is considered an expectorant, meaning it can make it easier for an individual to cough up material from the lungs and soothe a cough. Although science has not been interested in investigating these claims, osha has a long traditional use in treating colds.

Myrrh (*Commiphora* spp.) has a tradition of use for the common cold. Its essential oils are excellent decongestants and a myrrh plaster can be made to apply to the chest.[60] Myrrh also has antibacterial and anaesthetic properties.[61] Use it topically or as a tincture.

Astragalus *(Astragalus membranaceous)* is an herb with a reputation for strengthening the immune system. While it may not do much good once you have the symptoms of a cold, it is good to take during the fall to prepare your immune system for the onslaught of winter viruses. Or take it when the people around you are suffering from colds or other illness. It has several documented effects on the immune system.[62] Astragalus is usually taken as a liquid extract, or buy the root and try it in soup.

Both zinc and vitamin C are supplements that may help shorten the duration and intensity of a cold. Although there is some controversy among clinical trials, most trials have found that vitamin C supplementation of greater than 1 gram per day shortens the duration and the severity of cold symptoms, in both children and adults.[63] No trials have definitively determined an appropriate dose for vitamin C, but it is probably around 2 grams (2,000 milligrams) up to six times a day. Don't take it all at once, though. The body can process only 500–1,000 milligrams every two to three hours. If you get diarrhea, you are taking too much vitamin C and should cut back. Vitamin C may be especially beneficial to those who exercise a great deal. It appears that this group contracts more cold, which may be because physical stress uses up more vitamin C.[64]

Although zinc deficiency may suppress the immune system, whether zinc stimulates the immune system for individuals without deficiencies is still controversial. There is evidence that zinc can inhibit the binding of rhinoviruses to cells, thus inhibiting the infection process. A recent meta–analysis of the literature indicates that for adults, zinc is effective in reducing the duration and severity of cold symptoms. However, it must be taken at the first sign of a cold and in the form of zinc gluconate, 15 milligrams every two hours.[65] Not enough literature exists on other forms of zinc to make a determination of their value. A recent study at the Cleveland Clinic, however, found that zinc supplementation was not effective in treating cold symptoms in children from grades one to twelve.[66] More studies should be done before a conclusion is made regarding the use of zinc for children. Because zinc can cause nausea, don't take it on an empty stomach and don't take it for more than a week at a time.

A hot bath might be more than relaxing during a cold. Heat can actually stop the reproduction of the rhinovirus. A recent study found that incubating infected cells at 45°C (113°F) for twenty minutes prevented the virus from multiplying.[67] Although a 113°F bath may be a little too hot, sitting in a bath that is about 109°F for ten minutes may be quite therapeutic, especially if some essential oil is added to the water.

Also, while you have a cold, rest and let the cold run its course. Drink plenty of fluids to keep secretions of mucus thin. Eat whole foods to provide the body with nutrients and energy to deal with the cold. Use a humidifier to keep the nose and throat moist.

DANDRUFF

Dandruff, also called seborrheic dermatitis, is not necessarily an infectious disease but, rather, a type of dermatitis, or skin inflammation. It often becomes infected with the yeast *Malassezia furfur* or a tinea species of fungi (*see* athlete's foot section in this chapter). Dandruff appears as dry, flaking scales of skin and redness on the scalp and sometimes on the face, back, stomach, and folds of the body. It is more common in patients with Parkinson's disease and in the elderly. Psoriasis is a similar disease and may be confused with dandruff. Unfortunately, dandruff is usually a chronic ailment that lasts a lifetime.

Treatment for dandruff usually consists of shampoos that contain tar, zinc, pyrithione, or selenium. Sometimes the antifungal agent ketoconazole is administered, as are steroids. There are a few herbal treatments for dandruff, however. The Chickasaw Indians used to rub corn oil onto the scalp. Corn oil has anti-inflammatory activity and may reduce the amount of inflammation on the scalp.[68] Other oils may be of benefit—for example, flaxseed (linseed) and evening primrose oils, which impart essential fatty acids.

Use herbs with antifungal activity to limit infections of the scalp. Dilute tea tree or another antifungal essential oil in a carrier oil such as almond oil, and rub that on the scalp before bedtime. Antifungal essential oils useful for treating dandruff include:

Cedarwood
Citriodora
Eucalyptus
Manuka
Myrrh
Patchouli
Spikenard
Marigold
Tea Tree
Turmeric
Yuzu

Tea tree oil has demonstrated activity against yeasts that cause dandruff.[69] In the morning, wash the oil out and follow with an herbal rinse. Infuse apple cider vinegar with one of the antifungal herbs listed below (*see* chapter 9 for directions on making infusions), and pour this concoction over the head after washing your hair. These treatments can make a dandruff problem more manageable. Appropriate herbs for making the antidandruff hair rinse include:

Myrrh (*Commiphora* spp.)
Rosemary *(Rosmarinus officinalis)*
Sage *(Salvia officinalis)*
Thyme *(Thymus vulgaris)*

DIAPER RASH

Although diaper rash itself is not an infection, it can easily become infected if not taken care of properly. We typically think of diaper rash as affecting infants, but keep in mind that many adults, especially the elderly, have bladder problems and also wear a type of diaper. Diaper rash appears as reddened, swollen skin, sometimes with raised bumps or scaling and abrasions under the diaper-covered area. Because they hold wetness, diapers cause the skin to become overhydrated. This wet skin is more easily abraded when the diaper rubs against it. Take care when using diapers that they are well adjusted and that the tape from a disposable diaper does not cut into the skin. Urine and fecal matter in the diaper can also cause contact dermatitis. Always change diapers immediately.

Without complications, diaper rash usually will go away within two days. Yeast infections from diaper rash are a common complication, however, especially when antibiotic treatment is being administered for another condition. In the case of an infant, the mouth should also be checked for thrush. If this oral infection is present and the infant is breast-feeding, the mother may need to treat her nipples topically with an essential oil, such as lavender or tea tree oil, to control the infection. Diaper rash infections can also be bacterial, such as those caused by *Staphylococcus aureus*. If bacterial infection due to *S. aureus* is present in an infant under the age of one month, he may have acquired the bacteria from the hospital nursery, which should be promptly notified.

Follow proper procedures during a diaper change to ensure that infectious materials are not transmitted from person to person, especially in institutions such as day-care facilities and nursing homes.[70] Protect the changing area with a clean covering. The caregiver should make sure to wash the hands, to avoid passing infectious agents to the diaper wearer. The skin should be washed appropriately with water or some type of wipes. Diaper and wipes should be folded and disposed of properly. If cloth diapers are used, put them into an appropriate pail to await laundering. When diaper rash is present, a layer of zinc oxide should be applied to the skin for protection after it is cleaned. Afterward, the caregiver should again thoroughly wash hands, as well as the changing area.

When an infant has diaper rash, excess moisture is the main culprit. Allow the baby to be free of a diaper for as long as possible. Put down a thick towel in the crib and let the baby play in the crib without a diaper. Before you put a diaper back on, coat the diaper area with a zinc oxide paste. This will keep the moisture from soaking into the skin. There is no evidence that ointments containing vitamins work any better.

Take care whenever you put anything on a baby's skin, as allergics can be acquired easily. Lavender essential oil is usually safe to apply even to an infant's skin.[71] Dilute it slightly, perhaps half and half with a carrier oil, such as almond oil, and apply to the lesions on the skin. Chamomile oil or tea has healing and antimicrobial properties.[72] The tea can be used to clean the bottom and the essential oil can be diluted as for lavender and applied to the skin. Be aware that chamomile is a common allergen, and keep close watch on the baby's skin. For more severe diaper rash, try a dilution of tea tree oil. This oil has proven antimicrobial activity against a number of pathogens.[73]

Diarrhea

Besides being the primary side effect of antibiotic use, diarrhea is a disease in itself. In its severe form, it can—and often does—lead to death, especially in developing countries, where it often results from poor sanitation and contaminated drinking water, and where there is limited access to medical care. Those most at risk are infants and small children; the actual cause of death is dehydration. It can also be a serious concern in nursing homes in the United States. Diarrhea is defined by more numerous and liquid bowel movements. It can be an adverse reaction to various drugs, such as antibiotics, and can be caused by infection or by the toxins produced by bacteria. It may also result from eating spoiled food, drinking impure water, or ingesting an infectious agent from its presence on the hands. This can easily happen when you do not wash the hands properly after changing diapers, using the toilet, handling animals, and so on.

Bacterial infection of the intestines can be caused by *Escherichia coli, Staphylococcus aureus, Bacillus cereus,* or *Clostridium perfringens.* In the case of antibiotic use, the agent responsible for diarrhea is usually *C. difficile.* In the case of dysentery, which is accompanied by fever and bloody stools, the guilty organisms present can be *Shigella, Salmonella, Campylobacter, Yersinea,* or a toxin from the *E. coli* strain known as 0157:H7. Many parasites can cause diarrhea as well, including *Entamoeba histolytica, Giardia,* and *Trichomonas.* These protozoal parasites are present in some water supplies, especially in undeveloped countries.

Typically, diarrhea will come under control within five days. The single most dangerous effect of diarrhea is the loss of fluids. Replacing lost liquids is imperative. Drink plenty of fluids in the form of water, teas, juices, and vegetable broths. Electrolyte-replacement fluids, such as sports drinks, are also good. If diarrhea is accompanied by fever, severe abdominal pain, and tenderness or continues more than five days, it is important to see a physician. Pay attention to signs of dehydration as well—excessive thirst, dry mouth, decreased urination, and lethargy—especially in children. Chronic diarrhea that persists past five days may be due to a number of diseases, including malabsorption, or an inflammatory bowel disease, such as Crohn's disease. Diagnosis of the cause of chronic diarrhea should be made and the condition treated appropriately.

TREATING DIARRHEA WITH PROBIOTICS

During the course of diarrhea, stay away from high-fiber foods and caffeine, which stimulate the intestines. Reestablishing the normal bacterial environment in the intestinal ecosystem with probiotics can alleviate some types of diarrhea. Because diarrhea is a common side effect of radiation treatments and antibiotics, probiotics can also be used as a preventive measure and taken along with these treatments. Probiotics are living bacterial organisms found in yogurt, cheese, fortified milk, fortified soy milk, and sourdough bread. The most common probiotic organisms are *Lactobacillus acidophilus* and *L. bulgaricus,* both of which produce lactic acid and lactose. Lactic acid inhibits the growth of pathogenic bacteria, and lactose aids in digestion. Another bacterium, *Bifodobacterium,* binds to the lining of the intestine, preventing pathogenic bacteria from taking up residency there. *Bifodobacterium* is also adept at making B vitamins. When these beneficial bacteria enter the intestines, they can treat and prevent diarrhea.[74] The most important element to consider with probiotics, however, is how the manufacturing process affects them. As supplements in pill form, they are least likely to have the properties of living cultures. But yogurt and cheese have been shown to alter the intestinal flora in a positive way. This is probably the best source of probiotics, but be sure that the label reads "live cultures." The many beneficial effects of probiotics include:

- Helping prevent cancer
- Improving the immune system
- Preventing food allergies
- Preventing ulcers
- Reducing symptoms of arthritis
- Treating diarrhea
- Treating vaginal infections

Alternatively, there are prebiotics. Prebiotics are foods that can be eaten to promote the growth of "good" bacteria in the intestinal tract. The best prebiotic food is fructooligosaccharide, or FOS. This nondigestible carbohydrate is found in fruits, vegetables, and grains, as well as in commercial nutritional supplements.

Herbal Treatments for Diarrhea

Berberine has been shown to be effective in treating certain types of diarrhea.[75] Not only does berberine inhibit intestinal movement, but it also has antibacterial and anti-inflammatory effects. Herbs that contain berberine include bloodroot *(Sanguinaria canadensis)* and goldenseal *(Hydrastis canadensis)*. These herbs are usually taken as a liquid tincture one to three times a day. Do not take them if you are pregnant or nursing, because the effects on pregnancy and on the newborn are unknown.

Carob bean has a traditional use in treating diarrhea. One clinical study established that giving children carob bean juice during a bout of diarrhea curtailed the episode.[76] If carob juice is not available, use carob powder diluted in tea or juice a few times a day, or as often as every two hours. Pectin, a nondigestible fruit fiber, can also alleviate some types of diarrhea. Many commercial preparations contain pectin as well as a clay called kaolin, which absorbs some of the excess fluid of diarrhea.

Other herbal teas that may be beneficial in the treatment of diarrhea are red clover *(Trifolium pratense)*, flaxseed oil, guarana *(Paullinia cupana)*, red raspberry leaves, rose petal, shepherd's purse *(Capsella bursa-pastoris)*, bayberry bark *(Myrica cerifera)*, and wintergreen *(Gaultheria procumbens)*. The active ingredient of many of these herbs is probably tannic acid. Be sure to use the herb wintergreen, not the essential oil, which should not be ingested.

Chamomile tea can also be soothing to the intestines. One study showed that children with diarrhea who were given a commercial preparation containing apple pectin and chamomile extract recovered faster than did children given a placebo.[77] Drinking green tea may be beneficial as well. Green tea can inhibit the growth of many bacterial organisms associated with diarrhea.[78] Finally, some studies have shown that zinc can help prevent diarrhea and reduce the length of time of an episode. Zinc's effect is due to stimulation of the immune system in the case of diarrhea caused by infectious disease.[79]

EAR INFECTIONS

Although ear infections can occur in the inner, middle, or outer portions of the ear, it is the middle ear infections that seem most common. These infections of the middle ear are clinically referred to as otitis media. *Otitis* comes from the word *otic*, which concerns the ear; the ending *-itis* refers to an inflammation. *Media* is Latin for "middle." Infections of the inner ear are referred to as otitis interna and infections of the outer ear as otitis externa. This section will deal with otitis media, as otitis externa is essentially a skin infection and otitis interna is rare and should be dealt with by a physician.

ARE ANTIBIOTICS EFFECTIVE FOR TREATING EAR INFECTIONS?

Otitis media tends to be common in children and can cause severe pain in the ear. Many parents have fretted over the seemingly endless use of antibiotics to treat this condition. The decision as to whether to use antibiotics here is important because more antibiotics are prescribed for ear infections than for any other disease. In many cases it seems that as soon as a child finishes a course of antibiotics prescribed for an ear infection, the infection returns. Besides being used to treat acute cases of otitis media, antibiotics are sometimes prescribed in low dosages for prolonged periods as a means of preventing ear infections. Eliminating or decreasing antibiotic use for otitis media would have a significant effect on overall antibiotic use. For some time now, many people—physicians and parents alike—have questioned whether antibiotics actually provide any benefit for this condition. You may have heard from your physician that it is important to treat ear infections because the fluid buildup in the ear might interfere with hearing and language development. However, no research has supported this position. At one time, complications from ear infections such as mastoiditis, an infection of the skull bone behind the ear, and meningitis, an infection of the covering of the brain and spinal cord, were more common. But these complications do not seem to be as prevalent anymore, possibly due to changes in the bacteria themselves.

Many clinical studies have suggested that antibiotics have no benefit in treating otitis media, but this evidence hasn't been convincing enough for some. However, a recent clinical study has confirmed this suggestion by comparing a course of antibiotic treatment to no treatment. The conclusion from this study was that antibiotics provided no benefit over taking a watchful approach.[80] In this study, 240 children, from the ages of six months to two years, who were diagnosed with otitis media, were randomly assigned to receive the antibiotic amoxicillin or were given no treatment other than close watching to make sure the infection didn't worsen. In follow-up evaluations done at four and seven days and at six weeks, no significant differences were seen between the two groups. Thus, the use of antibiotics did not improve the symptoms of otitis media in this study.

The term *otitis media* actually refers to inflammation of the middle ear rather than to a bacterial infection, although the two often occur together. Infants and children tend to be more prone to otitis media because of the design of the eustachian tubes, or auditory canals. These tubes that connect the inner ear to the nose or throat are not fully formed in children, so fluid in the ear does not always drain properly into the nose, as it does in most adults. As fluid builds up, it causes pressure and pain on the eardrum that can lead to inflammation of the middle ear. It is this inflammation that is diagnosed as otitis media.

The fact that this condition is an inflammation rather than an infection may be one reason that antibiotics seem to provide no benefit. Sometimes, however, bacteria or viruses do grow in this environment, causing infection. But unless a fluid sample is taken, it is nearly impossible for a physician to know whether an infection exists, and, going further, to know whether an existing infection is caused by a bacterium or a virus. Typically, by the time a child turns six or seven, the auditory canal becomes large enough to allow good drainage and most children stop having chronic ear inflammation.

RISK FACTORS FOR
DEVELOPING OTITIS MEDIA

There are several identified risk factors for developing otitis media.[81] For instance, ear infections tend to run in families, so if you were prone to ear infections as a child, your son or daughter may also be prone to ear infections. Children at large day-care centers also tend to get more ear infections, presumably because they are exposed to more bacteria and viruses than are children who stay home or attend smaller day-care facilities. Children exposed to cigarette smoke also are at an increased risk for ear infections, as well as for respiratory problems. Breast-fed babies are less prone to ear infections probably because of immunity passed through breast milk. However, there is no guarantee, as breast-fed babies do get some ear infections. Ear infections also tend to follow a cold or to be associated with allergies. If these conditions are kept under control, the chance of ear infection can be reduced.

The number of physician's office visits for otitis media has greatly increased over the past ten years, for unknown reasons.[82] The result of this increase is a large increase in antibiotic-resistant bacteria, which in turn makes infections more difficult to treat. Infections of the ear can be caused by *Staphylococcus aureus* or *Moraxella catarrhalis*, but most are caused by *Streptococcus pneumoniae*. With the advent of penicillin, infections caused by *S. pneumoniae* became very easy to treat. However, the late 1980s brought the emergence of penicillin-resistant *S. pneumoniae*, and in the past fifteen years the number of penicillin-resistant *S. pneumoniae* in the United States has more than doubled. In Asia, occurrence of antibiotic-resistant strains of *S. pneumoniae* is as high as 70 percent of the occurrence of all *S. pneumoniae* reported; in the United States, resistant strains run as high as 25 percent. In day-care centers in the United States, occurrence is even higher, reaching 61 percent of all *S. pneumoniae* isolates.[83] These resistant bacteria are passed from one person to another and occur in particularly high percentages in children previously treated for otitis media. A recent study compared the number of antibiotic-resistant isolates of *S. pneumoniae* in the nasal passages of 120 pediatric patients before and after antibiotic treatment for otitis media. This number increased significantly after three to four days of treatment, putting these children at a greater risk of becoming infected with antibiotic-resistant strep. Of course, the risk that they would pass resistant bacteria on to others increased as well.[84] This becomes a serious problem, as antibiotic-resistant bacteria are far more difficult to treat than are nonresistant strains. The same resistant bacteria can cause pneumonia, sinusitis, bronchitis, and meningitis. There has been at least one report of death from meningitis attributed to infection by antibiotic-resistant bacteria in a child previously treated with antibiotics for uncomplicated acute otitis media.[85]

USE ANTIBIOTICS CAUTIOUSLY

Many physicians prescribe antibiotics because their patients (or in the case of ear infections, their patients' parents) expect them or even demand them. If circumstances convince you and your physician that antibiotics are necessary, make sure you use a narrow-spectrum antibiotic rather than a broad-spectrum antibiotic such as cefixime or ceftibuten. These broad-spectrum cephalosporin-type antibiotics are more expensive and are meant for more serious infections. Amoxicillin is the recommended antibiotic for treating ear infections, even for cases of recurrent otitis media.[86] It is important to remember that using a narrow-spectrum drug whenever possible will minimize the development of bacterial strains that are resistant to broad-spectrum antibiotics, thus saving the stronger drugs as effective resources for treating life-threatening diseases.

If your child is in general good health and no complications are suspected, suggest taking a watchful approach toward the condition. This means that you must be aware of any possible symptoms of a worsening case and you will seek further treatment if complications appear. Complications from ear infections include mastoiditis (infections in the skull behind the ear) and meningitis. Symptoms to look for include pain in the mastoid bone behind the ear, severe headache, and paralysis of the face. Ask your physician what other signs you should look for. In the majority of cases, taking antibiotics for otitis media has been shown to have no benefit over taking a watchful approach to the condition.[87]

In the United States, a ten-day course of antibiotics is typically prescribed for otitis media, even though few studies support this length of treatment. Clinical studies from Europe have been investigating the possibility of shorter courses of antibiotics for otitis media. A recent meta-analysis of the literature supports the use of a five-day antibiotic treatment for uncomplicated acute otitis media in children.[88] However, most of these studies used the antibiotic azithromycin rather than the preferred amoxicillin. More studies should determine whether shorter courses of amoxicillin can be successfully prescribed for control of otitis media when a bacterial infection is present.

Many people opt to delay treatment with antibiotics for twenty-four hours. This gives the condition time to resolve itself, as well as giving the immune system time to become activated. In most cases, pain from otitis media resolves in just a day, usually about as long as it takes to get to the physician. By waiting, the need for antibiotics may be eliminated. You can go ahead and get a prescription written, but save it. If pain and inflammation are still present after twenty-four hours, and you are still concerned, then consider having the prescription filled. In some parts of Europe, the standard procedure when treating ear infections is first to wait two days to see if the condition improves on its own. If symptoms persist, a five- to seven-day course of antibiotics is prescribed. [89]

ALTERNATIVE TREATMENTS FOR EAR INFECTIONS

There are alternatives to antibiotics for otitis media, and you will want to treat your child's pain. This pain results from pressure being put on the eardrum from fluid and inflammation in the middle ear. It typically lasts twenty-four hours with or without treatment. The American Academy of Pediatrics suggests using a warm compress against an older child's ear to relieve pain.[90] You can use a hot water bottle or a sock that has been filled with grain or flaxseed and warmed in the microwave.

Chewing gum relieves some pressure in the ear, but make sure the child is old enough not to swallow the gum (probably over age four). Gum sweetened with xylitol has shown some success in reducing the risk of ear infections.[91] Encourage your child to yawn in an effort to relieve pressure as well. Keeping the head propped up at night can promote draining of fluid from the eustachian tubes. An older child can use an extra pillow, but for a younger child, prop up the mattress with a wooden block or with books.

Herbs that can be used for otitis media include mullein *(Verbascum thapsus)* and garlic *(Allium sativum).* Mullein is a demulcent that can relieve congestion and inflammation. Compounds in mullein also have antibacterial, antiseptic, and pain-relieving properties.[92] Garlic, too, has both antibacterial and antiviral properties.[93] There are commercial ear drops available that contain these herbs. You can also make your own following the directions in chapter 9. A few drops of warm oil in the ear can provide great relief for a child feeling the pain of an ear inflammation.

When putting drops in a child's ear, make sure the oil is warmed; set the container in a bowl of warm water for a few minutes. Test the oil on your wrist as you would a baby's bottle. With the child lying on his or her side, put one to three drops of oil in the ear canal using a clean medicine dropper. Be careful to not get the dropper itself into the ear. Pulling slightly on the outer ear will help the oil run down into the ear canal. Also try massaging gently behind the ear. Use ear drops up to three times a day, but do not use drops if the eardrum is perforated.

A Personal Account

When my infant son began experiencing a series of ear infections and underwent antibiotic treatment, I decided to see if I could stop the cycle. The next time he had an ear infection, I told the pediatrician that I would rather not use antibiotics. A little worried, she asked me to take my son to an ear, nose, and throat specialist. After the specialist examined my son, he agreed with me. He said that many times antibiotics just don't seem to work, but that I should keep an eye on the infection and bring my son back if it didn't clear up soon. I took my son home and put mullein ear drops into his ears. A smile came across his face, and it was clear to me that this helped him feel much better. I continued this treatment a few times a day, and in three days the ear pain had cleared.

St. John's wort *(Hypericum perforatum)* has antiviral, antibacterial, and soothing qualities.[94] An oil infused with St. John's wort can be used as ear drops. Purchase this oil commercially or make your own from the tips of the branches including the flowers and leaves.

Many essential oils have soothing, antibacterial, and antiviral qualities that can be used in ear drops or massaged around the ear and lymph nodes. Lavender *(Lavandula officinalis)* and German chamomile *(Matricaria recutita)* are the most useful oils.[95] Dilute the essential oil in a vegetable oil base such as almond oil at a proportion of about half and half. Use a few drops of this warmed oil in the ear canal. Either of these oils can be massaged into the skin to soothe nerves and help promote sleep.

Because earaches are due to congestion in the eustachian tubes, using herbs that act as decongestants can be helpful. The mints, including peppermint *(Mentha piperita)* and catnip *(Nepeta cataria)*, have antiseptic and decongestant qualities that can help drain an inflamed ear.[96] Use peppermint as a tea and let the child drink as much as desired. Try mixing peppermint with chamomile as well. Chamomile has anti-inflammatory and slightly sedative qualities that may help relax a child in pain.

Although hot peppers such as cayenne *(Capsicum frutescens)* are known to have strong decongestant properties,[97] they may not be appropriate for children. Adults suffering from earache due to congestion can treat themselves to some hot salsa. As an alternative, hot pepper capsules are also available commercially.

If ear infections are recurrent, consider boosting the child's immune system. You can accomplish this with echinacea (*Echinacea* spp.) extracts as well as with vitamin C.[98, 99] Don't use the same dose you would use for yourself, however. Either use a formula made especially for children or use one quarter the adult dose of echinacea for children two to ten years old and half the adult dose for children over ten years old. For vitamin C, approximately 500 milligrams per day is a good dose for children. If a child develops diarrhea, it can mean that he or she is getting too much vitamin C, so cut back on the dose.

DECIDING WHETHER OR NOT TO USE ANTIBIOTICS

In the end, some ear infections do require treatment with antibiotics. The important thing to remember is to use antibiotics wisely, avoiding unnecessary (and dangerous) overuse. Keep the following points in mind when making decisions about whether or not to use antibiotics.

- Ask your physician whether antibiotics are absolutely necessary.
- Ask your physician about taking a shorter course of treatment, for three to seven days.
- Consider postponing antibiotic treatment for two or three days to see if the infection resolves itself.
- Use as narrow a spectrum antibiotic as possible, such as amoxicillin, rather than a broad-spectrum antibiotic, such as cefprozil or cefixime.

GINGIVITIS/PERIODONTAL DISEASE AND MOUTH SORES

Gum disease is one of the most prevalent chronic diseases in the United States. Painful, reddened gums that sometimes bleed are a sign of gingivitis, the first stage of periodontal disease. Periodontal disease is an infection of the gums by any number of oral bacteria—the long-term effect of plaque deposits on the teeth. Besides gingivitis, this plaque also causes dental caries, or cavities. Bacteria that give rise to periodontal disease include the *Actinomyces* and *Prevotella melaninogenica (Bacteroides melaninogenicus)*. These organisms also contribute to chronic sinusitis, chronic otitis media, and mastoiditis. They are a leading cause of bad breath. Sometimes gingivitis is caused by a yeast infection. When this is the case, the condition is sometimes called trench mouth. This is more common among people taking antibiotics for another condition. Gingivitis can also be caused by viruses.[100]

People at most risk of gingivitis are those with diabetes, pregnant women, and those with general illness or poor dental hygiene. Any type of irritation to the gums, such as is brought about by dentures and other dental appliances, can contribute to gingivitis. Hormonal changes also contribute to gingivitis, which is why it is prevalent during puberty. In fact, approximately 50 percent of high school students have gingivitis. Those with suppressed immunity such as AIDS patients and cancer patients are also more prone to gingivitis.

After the gums, the ligaments and bone become infected—the next stage of periodontal disease, and the main cause of tooth loss in adults. The most dangerous aspect of periodontal disease is that it is possible to inhale these organisms, leading to more serious infection that can spread to the lung, causing pneumonia or abscesses. In advanced periodontal disease, bacteria even invade the blood, reaching any of the organs. For this reason, periodontal disease is linked to heart disease, strokes, diabetes, and even premature birth.[101]

Penicillin is typically used to treat periodontal disease and oral pain, although prevention is certainly preferred. The American Academy of Periodontology suggests regular brushing and frequent visits to the dentist as the best ways to check periodontal disease.

At the first sign of gingivitis, take special care to brush the teeth and floss adequately. See a dentist for professional cleaning. You may want to ask a dentist or hygienist for instructions on proper brushing and flossing.

The key to inhibiting periodontal disease is to prevent plaque formation. Although regular brushing and flossing are usually enough, some people are more prone to plaque development and need a little extra help, such as mouth rinses. But there is little evidence that these rinses actually prevent gingivitis. Agents that act as antibacterials can reduce existing levels of plaque and prevent new plaque from forming. The American Dental Association's Council on Dental Therapeutics endorses the use of Listerine and chlorhexidine gluconate (Peridex) as dentrifices, or agents that reduce plaque. Chlorhexidine, though, can stain teeth. New research is focusing on the use of triclosan as a dentrifice, the same antibiotic agent that is found in most antibacterial soaps.

Listerine antiseptic, made by Warner-Lambert, was the first over-the-counter mouthwash. Introduced in 1914, it is named after Joseph Lister, a surgeon who pioneered such simple aseptic techniques as hand washing in surgery, which greatly decreased the death rate following surgery. Listerine is made from compounds found in essential oils: thymol, eucalyptol, methyl salicylate, and menthol.[102] Thymol, eucalyptol, and menthol all have proven antibacterial activity and are found in thyme *(Thymus vulgaris)*, eucalyptus *(Eucalyptus globulus)*, and peppermint *(Mentha piperita)*, respectively. Methyl salicylate has anti-inflammatory activity and is found in meadowsweet *(Filipendula ulmaria)* and willow *(Salix* spp.).[103] One Japanese study showed that chewing eucalyptus-containing gum three times a day had a significant effect on reducing plaque. Because of the strong flavor of eucalyptus, you might prefer to use it as a mouth rinse rather than as a gum.[104]

The American Dental Association advocates the use of sanguinarine compounds (Viadent) but notes that some studies do not support the use of sanguinarine as much as others.[105] Sanguinarine, an alkaloid found in bloodroot *(Sanguinaria canadensis)*, is becoming a common ingredient of both toothpastes and mouthwashes. It has proven activity against plaque and gingivitis. Its effectiveness as a mouthwash is better than as a toothpaste.[106]

Teas may be helpful in both preventing cavities and lowering the risk of gingivitis. Tests have found that green tea, black tea, and oolong tea can inhibit the growth of the oral bacteria that cause cavities. Furthermore, volunteers who rinsed with a solution containing oolong tea extract were found to have less plaque deposit on their teeth.[107]

Neem, or bark-containing sticks of *Azadirachta indica*, may inhibit plaque formation on the teeth. An extract from neem was able to prevent streptococci bacteria from sticking to a simulated toothlike surface, thus inhibiting the first step in plaque formation.[108] Chewing sticks, or meswaks, are used for teeth cleaning and oral health, particularly by Muslims. Brushing with the meswak stick improved study parameters measuring gingivitis, perhaps by increasing the amount of calcium and chloride present in the saliva. These benefits were lost after four hours, however, making continuous use necessary.[109]

Any of the antibacterial herbs can be made into a mouth rinse. Myrrh *(Commiphora myrrha)* has both antiseptic and anti-inflammatory properties. For this reason, it has traditionally been used as a gargle or mouth rinse to treat gum and mouth infections as well as sore throats. Sage *(Salvia officinalis)* is another good candidate for this type of use.[110]

INFLUENZA

A flu and a cold are often difficult to differentiate, but a flu is usually worse. Symptoms include a fever with chills, runny nose, cough, headache, and a feeling of malaise or tiredness. Influenza, or flu for short, is caused by influenza virus either A or B. Outbreaks of the flu tend to occur in epidemics in late fall or winter. Although the most acute symptoms usually subside within three days, symptoms such as weakness and coughing may persist for ten days.

Even though the flu is typically self-limiting, serious complications can arise in the very young or the elderly or those with a preexisting disease. These complications include pneumonia and, rarely, encephalitis and myocarditis. For these reasons, some health-care professionals as well as the Centers for Disease Control recommend influenza vaccinations. Influenza vaccinations must be received annually, as their contents change each year based on predictions of which strains of influenza will be prevalent. If this projected match is good, the vaccine is 70–90 percent effective in preventing influenza; when the match is not good, the rate of protection falls significantly.[111] These vaccinations can cause flu symptoms and their long-term side effects are not known.

Although physicians will usually recommend bed rest and drinking plenty of fluids for the flu, there are some pharmaceutical treatments available. Two antiviral drugs, rimantadine and amantadine, have been used to treat or prevent infections with influenza A but have not been used for influenza B. Side effects include nausea, upset stomach, headache, dizziness, and confusion. These drugs have proved to be of little use because of their lack of activity against influenza B and because of the development of viral resistance to these drugs.[112] A new class of antiviral drugs are the neuraminidase inhibitors such as zanamivir (Relenza) and oseltamivir (Tamiflu), which are effective against both influenza A and influenza B. These drugs act by preventing the attachment of the virus to surfaces in the body. Side effects of these drugs include nausea, diarrhea, and headache.[113] They are also costly treatments at $50 to $70 for a five-day course.

Many physicians, as well as the Centers for Disease Control (CDC), recommend vaccinating against the influenza virus. Although this may be a good idea for some, it is not without risks. Influenza vaccinations are different each year, based on a prediction of what viruses will be prevalent during the flu season. Because of this, protection is provided for just one year and revaccination is necessary each year. Side effects of this vaccine include many flulike symptoms—muscle aches, fever, and tiredness—as well as allergic reactions. Aspirin should not be taken by children or adolescents for these symptoms, as it may cause Reye's Syndrome, a life-threatening complication. The viruses for this immunization are grown on eggs, so an allergy to eggs is a contraindication for the vaccination. The flu shot provides an estimated 70 percent protection against getting the flu, less so in people over sixty-five years of age.

Elder *(Sambucus nigra)* has a tradition of use for the treatment of colds and flu and has stood the test of science. The flowers from this plant have demonstrated antiviral activity against both influenza types, A and B, as well as herpes simplex virus type 1. It also possesses anti-inflammatory activity. [114] A clinical study showed that a standardized elderberry extract, Sambucol, improved the symptoms of influenza with a complete recovery in two to three days, compared to a six-day recovery period for the group not receiving the herb. In this study patients were diagnosed with influenza type B.[115] Elder may act by stimulating the body's own interferon or by preventing attachment of the virus to the body's surfaces.

Licorice root has also demonstrated antiviral activity. When mice infected with lethal doses of influenza virus were treated with glycyrrhizin, an active component of licorice, they were protected from death due to the virus and had less lung damage than did mice treated with saline controls.[116]

As always, preventing an illness such as the flu is preferred. This might be accomplished by improving the immune system, specifically in the fall as flu season approaches. Several studies have shown that astragalus *(Astragalus membranaceous)* extracts can stimulate the immune system.[117] Use astragalus as an extract or add the root to soups.

Most treatments to relieve symptoms of the common cold are also applicable to influenza, so please refer to that section.

Lyme Disease

Lyme disease is a chronic condition that occurs as the result of a tick bite. The deer tick *(Ixodes dammimi)*, is a carrier for the pathogen *Borrelia burgdorferi,* which it transfers to warm-blooded mammals, including humans, with its bite. Although the symptoms of Lyme disease are highly variable, they typically progress in three stages.

At the first stage, a simple skin lesion appears three days to four weeks after the bite. This flat, red lesion slowly grows in size. Flulike symptoms, such as headache, fever, and chills, often accompany the lesion. Weeks to months later, the spirochete infects the blood or lymph fluid, causing more diverse symptoms. These symptoms may be additional skin lesions, joint and muscle pain, fatigue, and neurological impairment that includes paralysis of the face. Rarely, cardiac disease and meningitis are present. The third phase does not begin until months or even years later. It includes more severe skin, joint, and nervous system problems that become chronic. Nervous system afflictions are memory loss, mood changes, and sleep disturbances. The arthritis can be debilitating.

There are no reliable tests for confirming the presence of Lyme disease, so a diagnosis is made based on symptoms alone. This situation tends to precipitate overdiagnosis of the disease and an overuse of antibiotics for treatment of a disease that may not be there.[118]

The antibiotics tetracycline (doxycycline) and penicillin are used both to treat existing Lyme disease and to prevent the development of Lyme disease when a person knows he or she has been bitten by a tick. This is a highly controversial use of antibiotics. Studies have shown that prophylactic treatment has not halted the development of Lyme disease. It is preferable to wait a few weeks to determine whether symptoms arise; then take antibiotics if they do. Studies show that treating with antibiotics early in the course of the disease will prevent the later symptoms. It is hoped that in the future, more reliable tests will become available for detecting Lyme disease. No studies have been conducted to investigate treating Lyme disease with herbs. If you have concrete evidence of Lyme disease, antibiotics are the best choice. There are usually administered for four to six weeks. There are many herbs that can be taken along with antibiotics to support their action. For instance, by eating active yogurt culture, antibiotic damage to the intestinal tract can be minimized. Take garlic *(Allium sativum)* and echinacea (*Echinacea* spp.) to support the immune system. Vitamin B supplements may reduce nerve damage in the later stages of the disease.

A Personal Account

When the ethnobotanist and author Dr. James Duke was bitten by a tick, physicians could not be sure whether he had contracted Lyme disease. Due to the serious symptoms that the disease would cause several years later if he had indeed contracted it, he wanted to be safe and so opted to take antibiotics. However, to boost his immune system, he also took herbs as a complementary treatment. These herbs included echinacea (six 450 milligram tablets daily) and garlic capsules (equivalent to 1,200 milligrams of fresh garlic per day). Along with this, daily he drank a vitamin A concoction containing carrots and tomatoes. After three weeks he felt great and had no signs of Lyme disease. Was it the antibiotics, the herbs, or the combination? We'll never know for sure.

SCABIES

Scabies is a skin disease caused by the itch mite *Sarcoptes scabiei*, commonly called bed bugs—tiny mites on your skin that you can't even see! The main symptom of scabies is a severe itch, which is why it used to be called "the itch." These mites burrow into the surface of the skin, where they lay their eggs. Small vesicles are also common. The body parts that are most affected are the hands, wrists, armpits, genitalia, inner thighs, and elbows. Diagnosis is made by microscopic observation of the mites and their eggs.

Scabies outbreaks are more common where people live or interact in close proximity—for example, schools and nursing homes. Scabies is also endemic to underdeveloped countries. Immunocompromised patients, especially those with AIDS, are prone to scabies. More serious cases of scabies are often called crusted, or Norwegian, scabies; this form of the condition is usually much more difficult to treat.

Treatment for scabies is primarily a topical chlorinated hydrocarbon insecticide called lindane, a benzene hexachloride. This insecticide can be toxic to the blood and nervous system; for this reason, it cannot be used on children, pregnant women, or patients with a history of seizure disorders. Local skin irritation can also occur. Moreover, these insecticides are toxic to the environment, poisoning the soil and water. There is evidence of scabies resistance to lindane. Another drug, ivermectin, has been linked to increased numbers of deaths in nursing-home patients when used orally to eradicate scabies.[119] Less toxic treatments include the antiparasite drugs permethrin, crotamiton, sulfur, and benzyl benzoate. Systemic antibiotics are often used to prevent or treat secondary infections of the skin.

ALTERNATIVE TREATMENTS FOR SCABIES

There are no scientifically documented treatments for scabies. Because most standard treatments consist of a chlorinated hydrocarbon and as scabies is not a life-threatening disease, alternative treatments should be tried first. Historic treatments include buckbean or bogbean *(Menyanthes trifoliata)*, pansy *(Viola tricolor)*, and pine *(Pinus palustris)*.[120] An extract of aniseed *(Pimpinella anisum)* applied to the skin has also been used for scabies, as well as for other skin parasites. Try washing the skin with a strong tea made from the herbs. Dr. Jean Valnet recommends several essential oils for treating scabies, saying they will kill the mite in a matter of minutes.[121] Dilute the essential oils in a carrier oil and cover the infected area. Use a substantial amount of oil; besides its antipesticide activity, it will help suffocate the insects. Improvement may be seen only after several treatments. If you can stand the smell, rub the infected area with a clove of garlic *(Allium sativum)* or an oil that has had garlic soaked in it. If skin irriation develops, either discontinue use or try once more, but first coat the skin with a protective layer of olive oil. The following essential oils are effective for treating scabies:

Tea tree oil *(Melaleuca alternifolia)*
Clove oil *(Eugenia caryophyllata)*
Patchouli essential oil *(Pogostemon cablin)*

Lavender *(Lavandula angustifolia)*
Lemon *(Citrus limonum)*
Rosemary *(Rosmarinus officinalis)*
Orange flower*(Citrus aurantium)*
Cinnamon *(Cinnamomum zeylanicum)*
Mustard (*Sinapis* spp.)
Thyme *(Thymus vulgaris)*

SINUSITIS

Sinusitis is an inflammation or infection of the sinuses, which often follows a cold. When this inflammation produces enough swelling, it prevents normal drainage of the sinuses into the nose. (The sinuses are hollow cavities found in some bones.) Often, the sinuses become infected with bacteria, such as *Streptococcus pneumoniae, Staphlococcus aureus,* and *Moraxella catarrhalis.* It is the paranasal sinuses, located behind the face, that are usually affected by sinusitis. These sinuses include the frontal sinus, ethmoidal sinus, sphenoidal sinus, and maxillary sinus, all of which drain directly into the nasal cavity. They serve to produce mucus and provide resonance for speaking and singing. This is why the voice is often altered by sinusitis.

Depending on which sinus is affected, pain can be felt in the face over the cheeks, nose, or forehead or in the upper teeth. Computed tomography is sometimes used to determine the extent of sinusitis. Besides antibiotics, decongestants are part of the treatment. Sinusitis is particularly difficult to combat because the sinuses have very little blood flow; thus drugs in the bloodstream are not delivered readily to them. Nevertheless, antibiotics are frequently prescribed for sinusitis. In cases of chronic sinusitis, surgical treatments are sometimes used to drain the sinuses.

Many cases of sinusitis are the result of allergies. If this is a possibility, try to remove allergens from your house. Have your heating ducts cleaned out. Even foods can be allergens. Identifying all allergens that you are exposed to may help alleviate chronic sinusitis.

Herbal treatments for sinusitis are similar to those for bronchitis and even sore throat. You want to relieve congestion and pain as well as prevent bacterial growth. One good remedy is inhaling steam. Hang your head over a bowl of very hot water, then cover your head with a towel to keep in the steam. Keeping your eyes closed, breath in this steam through your nose, if possible. For a more potent effect, add a few drops of an essential oil with antimicrobial action. Tea tree, eucalyptus, lavender, peppermint, rosemary, and thyme oils are all fine candidates. Alternatively, add a handful of sage leaves to a pot of simmering water on the stove. This fills the air with sage constituents, which also have antimicrobial effects. As many times as possible during the day, stop by the pot and inhale deeply, to let the sage-filled steam enter the nose and lungs. Also try putting a warm herbal compress over the sinuses while lying down; this may relieve the pressure.

Both drinking and inhaling peppermint tea can do wonders for relieving sinus congestion. At the Celestial Seasonings tea plant in Boulder, Colorado, they keep their bags of peppermint leaves in a large closet separated from the other herbs, because the vapors are so strong. It is said that employees who are suffering from sinus congestion will occasionally enter that room to inhale the vapors and get some relief.

Sinusitis can cause headaches. A randomized, double-blind trial showed that rubbing Tiger Balm ointment on the temples relieved headache pain in as little as five minutes, with no adverse effects.[122] Tiger Balm is an ointment from China that contains menthol, camphor, cajeput oil, mint oil, clove oil, and cassia oil. It is typically recommended for relaxing sore muscles, but its components are mucus thinning as well.

Antibacterial herbs can be used directly in the nose to minimize the numbers of bacteria moving from the nose to the sinuses. Make a strong tea from goldenseal and, with an ear swab, rim the interior of the nostrils with the tea. This can also be done with an essential oil, such as lavender, tea tree, or rosemary, or try rinsing the nostrils. For other treatments for sinusitis, see the section on the common cold in this chapter.

SKIN INFECTIONS—MINOR

Infections of the skin are usually the result of its becoming dry and cracked or cut so that bacteria or fungi are allowed entry under the protective outer layer. Impetigo is the most common type of skin infection. It is highly contagious and can even be spread from one part of the skin to another. The bacteria that cause impetigo are usually *Staphylococcus aureus,* but they are sometimes the more dangerous group—A beta-hemolytic *Streptococcus* organisms. The part of the body most susceptible to impetigo is the face, around the mouth and nose. The only symptom is itching of the skin and small blister lesions or crusts, which are sometimes confused with contact dermatitis. More severe cases of impetigo, sometimes referred to as ecthyma, occur on the legs. Impetigo is diagnosed either by microscopic analysis for the presence of bacteria or by attempting to grow bacteria off a skin scraping in the laboratory. This method is similar to a throat culture and likewise takes forty-eight hours. Impetigo is usually treated with oral antibiotics.

Folliculitis is an infection of the hair follicles from any number of bacteria. One cause is bathing in hot tubs containing the bacterium *Pseudomonas aeruginosa.* If you suffer itching and burning near the hair follicles one to four days after using a hot tub, pseudomonas might be the culprit. Make sure you tell the owners of the hot tub, so they will add chlorine or bromine to the tub or change the water. These skin infections are rarely of concern, but they should be watched in case they worsen and infect deeper layers of skin.

A more serious type of folliculitis that affects the surrounding tissue is a boil, also called a furuncle. Boils typically are abscesses caused by infection of hair follicles by *Staphylococcus aureus.* An enlarged, sometimes yellow, rounded area of skin that is painful and tender may be the site of a boil. Usually a boil will gradually enlarge until it spontaneously opens and releases its contents of pus and dead tissue. This process takes from a few days to two weeks, and can be hastened by applying a warm herbal compress. Boils most often arise on the thighs, buttocks, back of the neck, or armpits. Even though the infection is generally self-limiting, most physicians will prescribe antibiotics. Those people who are prone to boils may be nasal carriers of *Staphylococcus aureus*. People who are immunocompromised or diabetic also may be prone to boils. Carriers of pathogenic nasal bacteria may benefit from topical treatment of the nostrils. Dust with goldenseal powder or rim the nostrils with a Q-tip soaked in lavender, tea tree, or rosemary oil twice daily for a few days.

Treating skin infections is relatively simple. Wash the skin with a strong tea made from an antimicrobial herb. These herbs are abundant and include goldenseal, myrrh, sage, rosemary, tea tree oil, and thyme.[123] Use whatever is most available to you. Essential oils diluted in carrier oils can be applied to the skin after cleansing. Place a warm poultice of goldenseal directly on the infected area or try applying tea tree oil diluted to 10 percent in a carrier oil. Taking echinacea or garlic internally can also help.

SORE THROAT

Also called acute pharyngitis, sore throats are especially common in children, and their management remains controversial in the medical community. Studies support the belief that antibiotics rarely change the course of a sore throat.[124] A recent study examined the effects of prescribing antibiotics for self-limiting diseases such as sore throats and found that one not-trivial side effect was the medicalization of minor illnesses. By giving antibiotics, physicians were encouraging patients to continue to return for every minor illness they contracted.[125] When antibiotics were prescribed, the patients' belief in them was confirmed, resulting in a long-term effect of more antibiotic use.

Most sore throats are caused by viruses, including mononucleosis, influenza, and viruses that cause the common cold. However, there are bacterial causes as well, the most widely known of which is *Streptococcus*, but these causes also include *Diphtheria*, and *Neisseria gonorrhoeae*, albeit rarely. The type of *Streptococcus* responsible for acute, bacterial pharyngitis is group A beta-hemolytic strep (GABHS). At one time, a sore throat caused by GABHS often progressed to abscesses on the tonsils, septicemia, and sometimes rheumatic fever and glomerulonephritis, or kidney problems. These events rarely happen now, and whether that is due to the use of antibiotics or to a change in virulence of the GABHS can never be known. A recent literature review, however, reports that the incidence of rheumatic fever has been declining for at least one hundred fifty years, beginning long before antibiotics were even used.[126] Although rare in developed countries, rheumatic fever remains a problem in developing countries. Those who have had rheumatic fever are more prone to a recurrence, and are generally treated long term with antibiotics as a preventive measure, sometimes for life if heart damage is serious.[127] Another side effect of strep throat—scarlet fever—has become a relatively benign disease that rarely ends in mortality, as it once did.[128] Scarlet fever results when the toxins produced from the bacteria have spread through the body, causing a rash on the trunk and neck.

A Personal Account

Brian came down with a bad cold and sore throat and went to the doctor for treatment. When antibiotics were recommended he didn't question the prescription, but went home and took them. They didn't agree with him, and when his cold symptoms worsened, he returned to his HMO. This time he saw a different doctor and again received antibiotics. Too sick to question, he began taking those as well as his previous prescription. He came down with a serious case of diarrhea and within three days was so dehydrated that he could not move. A friend who came to visit took him to the emergency room. He was admitted to the hospital and stayed there for three days while they rehydrated him. It took more than a year of probiotic treatment and a careful diet for him to recover fully.

The most serious side effect of strep throat is the development of rheumatic fever. This is the most important reason to treat a strep throat and other strep infections with antibiotics. Rheumatic fever can develop two to three weeks after strep throat infection and involves inflammation of the heart and joints. The disease is typically more serious in children than in adults. However, the risk of contracting rheumatic fever after a serious case of strep throat is only 3 percent.[129] The disease usually resolves itself, but the most serious aspect of rheumatic fever is the incidence of valvular heart disease, which can lead to death. Another serious consequence of strep infection is acute poststreptococcal glomerulonephritis, or kidney disease. This too is quite rare, and is caused only by a very specific strain of *Streptococcus*.

Although sometimes strep throat is without symptoms, it typically involves a sore throat, headache, abdominal pain, fever, body aches, and nausea.[130] The tonsils and the back of the throat often appear red, swollen, and speckled with white spots of pus. Symptoms usually appear one to three days after exposure to group A strep. Because these symptoms also occur with other respiratory illnesses, they are not specific for strep throat. The conventional method for diagnosing streptococcal infection is with a throat culture. Unfortunately, nothing can differentiate an acute streptococcal infection from a streptococcal carrier state with a viral infection. Antigen detection tests, also referred to as "quick tests," can also be performed to detect the presence of group A beta-hemolytic strep, although they are not very sensitive and negative results must be backed up by negative cultures. If strep is present, the preferred treatment is to give penicillin by muscular injection. However, oral treatment is usually given instead for ten days. Studies show that even when penicillin is given up to nine days after the onset of illness, it is still effective in preventing rheumatic fever.[131] Thus, performing the proper tests to confirm the cause of disease does not put the patient at risk, but does prevent the unnecessary use of antibiotics. If a family member or someone you are in close contact with comes down with strep throat, you too should be tested at the first sign of a sore throat, as strep is highly contagious.

Some people are carriers of strep, meaning that they harbor the strep bacteria in their throats at low numbers. The amount of bacteria is not enough for these people to become ill, but is enough for them to pass the bacteria along to other people. However, carriers of strep may also often come down with strep throat . A throat culture can detect carriers of the disease.

There are many natural treatments for non-strep sore throats. First, it is important to rest, avoid refined sugar, and drink as much liquid as possible. The next line of treatment should be to support the immune system with herbs and vitamins, such as echinacea and vitamin C. Next, fight the infection by gargling and rinsing the mouth with a tea made from an herb with antibiotic activity. Gargling puts the medicine right where it is needed, at the back of the mouth. Alleviate the painful symptoms, such as inflammation, with soothing herbs and herb tea.

A Personal Account

Carol suffered quite frequently from sore throats, so often that she took antibiotics four times in one winter. Becoming concerned about frequent usage of antibiotics, she sought another solution to her sore throats, even though the diagnoses were often strep. The next time a sore throat arrived, she gargled every four to six hours with a strong tea made from goldenseal. Although the taste was not pleasant, the sore throat was relieved after a day, negating the need for antibiotics. Carol was relieved, and this time her sore throat did not come back for at least a year. Now, whenever she feels the slightest tingle of a sore throat, she uses a lozenge that contains zinc, vitamin C, goldenseal, and echinacea. So far this regimen has prevented symptoms from developing.

Goldenseal *(Hydrastis canadensis)* has a long history of topical use for skin disorders; it contains hydrastine and berberine, both with strong antibiotic activity. Berberine has demonstrated activity against *Streptococcus* and other bacteria.[132] Goldenseal works best when it comes in direct contact with bacteria, thus the best way to use it is as a gargle or a lozenge. Honey can improve the taste and has antibiotic qualities as well. There are zinc lozenges that contain goldenseal. Use these at the first sign of a sore throat—they can prevent further development. Do not use goldenseal if you have high blood pressure or if you are pregnant or nursing.

Other herbs containing berberine are Oregon grape *(Berberis aquifolium),* barberry *(Berberis vulgaris),* and goldthread *(Coptis chinensis).* *(See* chapter 8 for more information.)

Myrrh (*Commiphora* spp.) has both antibacterial and anti-inflammatory effects. This double action is important, as a sore throat is also an inflamed throat. Myrrh also acts as an analgesic to relieve the pain of a sore throat.[133] Good toxicity studies are not available for myrrh. Internal use is not recommended, but as a gargle it should be harmless.

Thyme *(Thymus vulgaris)* extracts, especially the volatile oils thymol and carvacrol, possess antibacterial activity.[134] When extracted in honey, the combination makes an effective and tasty syrup to be taken for a sore throat. Honey itself is soothing and has antibiotic properties. Do not use undiluted thyme oil, however; it can be toxic. Instead, extract fresh thyme from your garden by putting it in honey. Leave it in the sun for two weeks and keep the concoction on hand for sore throats, colds, and upper-respiratory-tract infections (*see* chapter 9). Brew a strong tea from the leaves of thyme and use as a gargle. Sometimes I make these medicines in summer and put small amounts in ice-cube trays to save for the winter months.

The bark of slippery elm *(Ulmus fulva)* can relieve a sore throat. Drink it as a tea, suck on a stick of slippery elm, or take lozenges containing the herb. Its soothing action is due the presence of mucilage, which lubricates the throat.[135] Herbs that are soothing to the throat and mucous membranes are called demulcents. Besides slippery elm, acacia, barberry, horehound, licorice, marsh mallow, and mullein can be brewed as teas to treat sore throats.

Tea tree oil has well-documented antibacterial activity, including activity against *Streptococcus*.[136] Although the taste is not pleasant, you can dilute it by adding a few drops to water or tea and then use it as a gargle. Do not swallow tea tree oil, though, as it is known to cause central nervous system toxicity in large amounts. As for any herb, it is good to first apply a drop to the skin to check for allergic reaction.

Turmeric *(Curcuma longa)* contains anti-inflammatory agents that relieve swelling in the throat. It also has antimicrobial properties that can help fight infections.[137] Make a gargle solution with one teaspoon of turmeric in a cup of warm water.

Ginger *(Zingiber officinale)* also has both anti-inflammatory and antimicrobial properties.[138] The best way to use ginger is to pour hot water over a few slices of fresh gingerroot and let it steep. Add maple syrup as a sweetener. Drinking this tea can help alleviate many symptoms of a sore throat as well as those of a cold.

If you can tolerate it, cayenne *(Capsicum frutescens)*, along with other hot peppers, contains capsaicin, which is a pain reliever, an anti-inflammatory agent, and an antibacterial.[139] Gargle with a tea made from cayenne with lemon juice to help relieve the pain associated with a sore throat.

Ulcers—Stomach/Peptic

The stomach is not a place where bacterial disease would have been suspected even just ten years ago. Because of its acidic environment, it is a hostile place for most living things, including bacteria. However, we now know that a tenacious bacterium called *Helicobacter pylori* can live in the stomach. It may lead to gastritis, peptic ulcers, and even stomach cancer. In fact, scientists now suspect that *H. pylori* may even be the source of diseases outside the gastrointestinal tract. Once thought to be related only to excess acid secretion in the stomach, ulcers are now recognized to have three sources. Besides excess acid secretion in the stomach, chronic use of nonsteroidal anti-inflammatory drugs (NSAIDs) and infection with the bacterium *H. pylori* are known causes of ulcers. When used for long periods, NSAIDS such as aspirin can produce ulcers not only in the stomach but also in the intestines. The bacterial source of ulcers is not well understood, but a correlation has been made between the presence of *H. pylori* in the stomach and the incidence of ulcers.

H. pylori is also associated with chronic gastritis. Gastritis causes discomfort in the upper abdomen and indigestion. Although most people infected with *H. pylori* will not experience gastric problems, such gastric irritation, when it occurs, can then develop into ulcers. These may bleed, causing a darkening of the stools. Ulcers typically heal over but tend to recur. They produce a burning pain and can be accompanied by a hungry feeling.

Patients diagnosed with this type of ulcer usually receive antibiotic treatment, which resolves the situation in the majority of cases. Antibiotic treatment usually involves the use of several antibiotics at a time, however, which results in severe side effects that can interrupt daily activities. Patients are subject to recurrences of *H. pylori* infection as well. And there are now antibiotic-resistant strains of *H. pylori*. If a patient has been treated once for *H. pylori*–induced ulcers, care should be taken to avoid reinfection by keeping the digestive tract healthy.

Past medical advice for patients to eat bland and restrictive diets is no longer in vogue. A well-balanced diet and meals at regular intervals are still recommended, as is eating a less acidic diet. Smoking can slow the rate of ulcer healing and is discouraged. Many times ulcers worsen with stress, and abdominal pain is felt most during those periods. Current treatment for ulcers accompanied by *H. pylori* is prescription of a proton pump inhibitor, such as comeprazole (Prilosec), along with two antibiotics.[140] Resistant strains of *H. pylori* are also becoming more common, making treatment more difficult.[141] *H. pylori*–related ulcers should not be taken lightly, as some evidence suggests that they are also related to gastric cancer.[142]

To minimize the risk of ulcers, first make sure your diet is rich in fiber and whole foods. Eat plenty of foods high in vitamin C, as vitamin C has been shown to inhibit the growth of *H. pylori*. In fact, the administration of 5 grams of vitamin C per day for four weeks to patients diagnosed with *H. pylori* infection showed a high cure rate with no side effects.[143] Epidemiological studies also indicate that high levels of vitamin C in the diet can reduce the risk of stomach cancer.[144] These effects could be due to the antioxidant quality of the vitamin.

The use of probiotics may also decrease the risk of ulcers. Some of these live bacterial cultures found in yogurt can inhibit the growth of *H. pylori; Lactobacillus salivarius* is particularly effective.[145] They may also displace *H. pylori* from the stomach lining. No human studies to date have examined the role of probiotics in controlling *H. pylori* infection.

The goals of treating stomach ulcers or gastritis are to eradicate the infection and to soothe the stomach and protect it from damage. Herbs and mild treatments can accomplish both of these. Herbs containing mucilaginous properties can coat the stomach lining, protecting it from damage. These herbs include marsh mallow *(Althaea officinalis)*, meadowsweet *(Filipendula ulmaria)*, and slippery elm *(Ulmus fulva)*.[146] Herbalists call these demulcents. The most thoroughly studied demulcent, however, is licorice *(Glycyrrhiza glabra)*.

The activities of licorice that are beneficial toward healing an ulcer include anti-inflammatory, antibacterial, and soothing properties. Because of these, licorice has a long history of use in healing ulcers.[147] Clinical and laboratory studies have documented this use as well, with several of them using a derivative of glycyrrhetinic acid called carbenoxolone.[148] Licorice can be used as a tea made from the root or as an extract. Licorice can produce many side effects, however, involving water retention, and should be avoided especially by people with an existing cardiovascular disorder. Look for a licorice product that has had the glycyrrhetinic acid removed or is referred to as deglycyrrhizinated licorice (DGL). This type has fewer side effects. One way licorice may work is by affecting the metabolism of prostaglandins, rasing the concentration of those that promote mucus secretion and cell growth to aid in healing.[149] Unsaturated fatty acids, such as arachidonic and linoleic acids, may be protective for the same reasons.[150]

Calendula *(Calendula officinalis)*, also called pot marigold, is another traditional treatment for gastritis and ulcers. This flower has anti-inflammatory, antibacterial, and soothing properties, as well as immune-stimulating activity.[151] Clinical trials have also shown it to be effective.[152] Use calendula in a tea or as a liquid tincture.

Some antibacterial herbs are especially useful for treating ulcers: garlic *(Allium sativum)* and berberine-containing herbs such as goldenseal *(Hydrastis canadensis)*. Garlic contains anti-bacterial effects including activity against *H. pylori.* [153] Epidemiological studies have shown that consumption of garlic is related to rates of infection by *H. pylori* lower than the rates of infection for people who don't consume garlic.[154] Although it is difficult to make a suggestion as to how much garlic can be beneficial, consider using it liberally in your food. Goldenseal has a tradition of being used to treat gastritis and ulcers. Its active ingredient, berberine, has antibacterial activity including toward *H. pylori.*[155] It can be used as a liquid extract. The ethnobotanist James Duke suggests using shrub yellow root *(Xanthorhiza simplicissima)* tincture, which also contains berberine.[156]

Although herbs from around the world have been suggested as ulcer treatments, recent studies point to the effectiveness of certain herbs that may be more common in our country. These include black tea *(Camellia sinensis),*[157] turmeric *(Curcuma longa),*[158] and holy basil *(Ocimum sanctum)*.[159] Try including more of these herbs in your diet.

In Japan, the herb *Rabdosia trichocarpa* is a common home remedy for stomach complaints. Studies have shown that this herb has antimicrobial activity against *H. pylori.* No human studies have been done to date.[160]

Note: Sometimes heart problems can have symptoms similar to those of an ulcer. If you have a history of heart problems, see a doctor if you have pains in the chest and stomach area.

URINARY TRACT INFECTIONS (UTI)

Infections can happen anywhere in the urinary tract, from the urethra to the kidneys. The urethra is the canal that moves urine from the bladder to the outside of the body. Besides the urethra, the urinary tract consists of the bladder, ureters, and kidneys. Inflammation and infections usually begin at the opening of the urethra

TABLE 12. TERMINOLOGY FOR INFECTIONS OF THE
URINARY TRACT

Medical Term	Type of Infection
Cystitis	Infection or inflammation of the bladder that holds the urine
Pyelonephritis	Infection or inflammation that has spread to the kidney
Ureteritis	Infection or inflammation of the ureter, the tube carrying urine from the kidneys to the bladder
Urethritis	Infection or inflammation of the urethra, or tube carrying urine out of the body

and then move up, causing cystitis in the bladder and nephritis in the kidneys. As the infection moves up, it becomes more serious. Urinary tract infections are much more common in women than in men, probably owing to the anatomical proximity of the urethra to the anus. Infections are especially common in older women, because of other bladder problems.

Uncomplicated urinary tract infections usually result from infection by the bacteria *Escherichia coli*, which is a common inhabitant of the bowel. They become complicated when another problem exists, such as kidney stones, malformations of the urinary tract, spinal cord injury, or a compromised immune system. These infections are typically treated with trimethoprim-sulfamethoxazole. Resistance to this antibiotic doubled from 1992 to 1996.[161] Resistance to other antibiotics has increased in urinary tract pathogens as well. Other organisms that can cause urinary tract infections include *Candida staphyloccocus, Enterobacter,* and *Klebsiella.* Urinary tract infections can be acquired in hospitals, especially through the use of catheters. People with diabetes tend to have more urinary tract infections, as do hospitalized patients. Urinary tract infections also can be sexually transmitted, and some people are more susceptible to these infections for unknown reasons.

If a lower urinary tract infection does not resolve, it can move up the tract, infecting the bladder and possibly the kidneys, where it can cause kidney damage. If the infection travels into the blood, additional complications may arise. Those who have had a urinary tract infection are more susceptible to them. Patients need to be aware of the symptoms so that a physician can be notified if the infection recurs.

Sometimes there are no symptoms; when there are, they may include pain and a burning sensation when urinating, a frequent and pressing urge to urinate, and passing blood in the urine. In men, a discharge from the urethra is common. Signs that the infection may be worsening are fever and chills, nausea, vomiting, and lower-back pain. The diagnosis is made simply by microscopic examination of the urine for the presence of bacteria and white blood cells.

Postmenopausal women often have more UTI because their lower estrogen levels cause an increased pH in the vagina. This change in pH allows different bacteria to colonize the vagina. The beneficial lactobacilli prefer an acid pH.[162] If you do not wish to take hormones orally, estrogen or progesterone creams or suppositories can put the hormone directly where it's needed. Occasional douching with a dilute vinegar solution can be helpful as well.

For people who have recurrent urinary tract infections, drinking lots of fluids at the first sign of an infection can ward it off—the fluid dilutes the bacteria present and flushes them from the body. Take these steps to keep the urinary tract healthy and lessen the risk of infection. Drink plenty of fluids. Do not hold urine when you have the urge to urinate. After a bowel movement, women should wipe from front to rear to keep bowel bacteria at a distance. Wear cotton underwear, rinse off soap well in the shower, and urinate after sexual intercourse. Using a pure glycerine soap can decrease the amount of inflammation in the area. A compress of witch hazel may also provide relief.

Once a folk remedy, cranberry juice has now gained the respect of the medical community for the treatment of UTI. Research has shown that cranberry juice contains a compound that blocks the bacteria from sticking to the lining of the urinary bladder. The first step in infection is the adhering of bacteria to a surface. One controlled clinical study showed that women who drank ten ounces of cranberry juice daily had fewer urinary tract infections than did women who had only a vitamin C drink.[163] Drink a glass of cranberry juice daily at the first sign of infection, or drink it on a regular basis if you are prone to UTI. Be careful not to ingest too much sugar, however; avoid cranberry juice cocktails, which are highly sweetened. Drinking cranberry juice may be the best way to gain the benefits of the fruit, as the quality of cranberry pills varies greatly. Blueberries, which are closely related to cranberries, contain the same compound. They, too, can lower the incidence of urinary tract infections.

An herb that is related to the cranberry is uva-ursi *(Arctostaphylos uva-ursi)*, also called bearberry. It has been used traditionally for urinary tract infection, although no studies have documented its effectiveness. It has been shown to have antimicrobial activity toward bacteria that cause urinary tract infections.[164] This activity is probably due to the quinone arbutin present in the leaves of the plant. Take uva-ursi as an infusion of the leaves or as a liquid extract. This herb is not recommended for long-term use in preventing urinary tract infections, however; the side effects include nausea, vomiting, ringing in the ears, and shortness of breath.

Chamomile has antimicrobial and anti-inflammatory properties that may alleviate symptoms of urinary tract infections (*see* chapter 8 for more information). One study treated patients with cystitis (an infection of the lower urinary tract) with the antibiotic Cotrimoxazol (trimethoprim-sulfamethoxazole). Half of the women also had a daily sitz bath with a chamomile extract. These women experienced relief of symptoms faster than did the women who did not have the chamomile baths.[165] Feel free to try this technique with or without antibiotics for infections of the lower urinary tract. The use of probiotics as vaginal suppositories has also been successful in treating recurrent urinary tract infections.[166] If you experience frequent UTI, you may also want to try immune-enhancing herbs such as astragalus and echinacea.

VIRAL INFECTIONS

Treatment of viral infections is often disappointing, and much research is dedicated to finding and developing antiviral drugs. Viral infections run from relatively benign (colds) to severe (HIV, viral meningitis). There are signs now that both herpes simplex virus (HSV) and human immunodeficiency virus (HIV) are developing resistant strains owing to treatment with current antiviral drugs. Some of the ongoing research is now focusing on herbs that have antiviral activity.

Several herbs have been shown to have activity against the herpes simplex virus. In one experiment, extracts from the herbs *Geum japonicum, Rhus javanica, Terminalia chebula,* and *Syzygium aromaticum,* more familiarly called cloves, exhibited activity against herpes simplex virus type 1 (HSV-1). In this experiment, mice were given a water-based extract from each herb alone, three times daily for seven successive days, after being inoculated with the HSV-1 virus. The herb extract delayed the appearance of skin lesions and death in these mice. When administered along with the antiviral drug acyclovir, these herbs showed improved antiviral activity compared with acyclovir alone. These herbs may act differently from acyclovir in inhibiting HSV-1 and thus may be more potent when used with acyclovir for severe infection.[167] Skin lesions can be induced in mice who are carriers of HSV-1 by treatment with ultraviolet light. When mice were pretreated with any of these herbs, the formation and severity of skin lesions were decreased after ultraviolet light induction. These herbs have also inhibited HSV-1 infection of cells in culture.[168]

These same herbs also showed antiviral activity against cytomegalovirus (CMV), which is a type of herpesvirus that is the cause of some birth defects in the babies of infected women. The virus also causes pneumonia. In one study mice were given oral, water-soluble extracts of *Geum japonicum, Terminalia chebula,* or *Syzygium aromaticum* three times daily. After one day of treatment, the mice were infected with CMV. After another sixteen days, the mice treated with any of these herbs had less of a viral load in their lungs than did mice not treated with the herbs. These herbs were also able to inhibit the replication of CMV in cells in culture.[169]

The Coxsackie viruses cause a number of diseases in humans, the most serious of which is viral heart disease. Treatment with astragalus *(Astragalus membranaceus)* injections prevented viral heart disease in mice when they were inoculated with the Coxsackie virus. In cell culture, astragalus inhibited the replication of the virus.[170] Although these results are preliminary, astragalus may prove to be an effective treatment or preventive measure for viral heart disease in the future.

Assaying plant materials for activity against HIV-1 is an active area of investigation in the fight against AIDS. Schizandra has shown some effectiveness against the AIDS virus. Compounds called gomisins found in *Schizandra chinensis* have been found to inhibit the reverse transcriptase enzyme from HIV-1. After repeated use in cell culture, however, the virus developed resistance to the schizandra extract.[171] Nigranoic acid, a triterpenoid from *S. spaerandra,* also inhibited the reverse transcriptase enzyme of HIV-1.[172]

Other plant parts that have demonstrated anti-HIV-1 activity include seeds from *Areca catechu* and bark from *Eugenia jambolana, Saraca indica,* and *Terminalia arjuna.* Their activity was directed against the HIV-1 protease enzyme. This enzyme is necessary for the formation of the virus.[173] To date, none of these viral treatments has been approved for human use. With ongoing laboratory experimentation, clinical studies may begin soon. Until then, it is not recommended to self-treat with any herbs for viral diseases, other than the ones listed in the sections on cold sores, colds, and flu.

WARTS

A wart is a mass of tissue that grows slowly from the skin, and can take on an assortment of sizes and shapes. Warts are most common on children and the elderly. Usually, skin warts are caused by a virus called human papillomavirus, of which there are many varieties. This virus makes the cells in the epidermis overgrow and push upward, forming the lump we call a wart. This is not a cancerous growth and will not invade surrounding tissue or cause problems in other areas of the body; however, it can be confused with more dangerous disorders that should be ruled out by a physician. The appearance of warts varies greatly, depending on the particular virus. They may be fingerlike projections from the skin or can remain flat. A main characteristic of warts is that they lack the typical skin lines.

Warts can appear anywhere on the body and are usually harmless. Most will go away within a few months, but they can block passages if they grow in the nose or ear. When they appear on the foot, they are referred to as plantar warts. These warts often affect the sole of the foot and can cause pain when walking. Some are easily removed by liquid nitrogen or agents that slowly dissolve the wart. Surgical removal is another treatment option, but warts often reappear.

Warts on the genitalia can be contagious. These types of warts are caused by a sexually transmitted virus called herpes simplex 2 (HSV-2), and they are associated with an increased risk of genital cancers. Patients can be infected with herpes and not show any symptoms, although they are still able to transmit the disease. The skin lesions associated with herpes are groups of small vesicles that are usually painful. These lesions then become crusted after about a week. Genital herpes is usually treated with the antiviral medication acyclovir. This drug is now being used so much that many people in the medical community are concerned that the herpesviruses will mutate to become resistant, just as bacteria have done in response to antibiotics.

There are several safe and effective natural treatments to hasten the disappearance of a wart. The most widely known is greater celandine *(Chelidonium majus),* which grows wild in many parts of the United States where there are forests. It contains a yellow-orange juice that you can squeeze out directly onto the wart.[174] The juice is irritating, however, and should not be allowed to come into contact with other parts of the skin. It probably acts similarly to commercial products and burns off the wart. No clinical research has been done on this herb.

Bloodroot *(Sanguinaria canadensis)* has more of a reputation for fighting gingivitis, but it is also used for warts. This herb is also known as red Indian paint, and it grows wild in the eastern United States. A powder derived from bloodroot was used by European settlers to treat skin warts, polyps of the nose, and eczema. This herb most likely also provides a certain amount of anesthesia to inflamed areas of skin.[175]

One herbal treatment for genital herpes is American mandrake root, or mayapple *(Podophyllum peltatum)*. The mayapple contains a compound called podophyllin, which is very toxic. Because of its toxicity to the skin, it readily removes warts, both common and genital.[176] It is best to use mayapple only with guidance from an experienced herbal practitioner.

Over-the-counter treatments for warts involve agents that are keratinolytic, meaning that they can dissolve the buildup of skin that makes the wart. The most common of them is salicylic acid, or aspirin. For a simple home remedy, apply a layer of olive oil on the wart and place an aspirin on top. Instead of aspirin, you can use a salicylate-containing herb, such as willow bark or meadowsweet extract. After applying the aspirin or herb extract, cover the wart with tape or a bandage. Other herbs to try for warts include papaya *(Carica papaya)*, prickly poppy (*Argemone* spp.), the sap from fendler spurge (*Euphorbia* spp.), and willow *(Salix alba)*. An easier method for treating warts might be to apply an essential oil with antiviral properties, such as lemon, lavender, tea tree, or geranium oil. Because research is lacking in the area of wart treatment, we tend to rely on these traditional treatments, especially as warts are a benign and self-limiting condition.

WOUND TREATMENT

One important purpose of the skin is to protect the body by preventing the entrance of pathogens that can cause infection. If the skin is not kept intact, it cannot perform its function. Anytime the epidermis is abraded, the skin—and likewise the rest of the body—becomes more prone to infection. It is the normal skin flora of streptococci or staphylococci species that will typically infect the skin, given the chance. The key to preventing infections is to keep the skin healthy. When it does become damaged, support its healing. Healing involves several stages: movement of basal cells of the epidermis to cover the dermal layer of skin, manufacture of proteins to help fill in the gap, and growth of new skin cells to cover the abrasion. The time it takes for a minor abrasion to heal is about two days. Deeper abrasions that go into the dermal layer of skin take longer and involve more steps in the healing process. These steps include formation of a blood clot, inflammation, movement and growth of epithelial cells under the scab, growth of fibroblasts, and scar formation. Before treating a wound, wash it well, making sure that no foreign elements are stuck in it. Various herbs can then be used to promote healing as well as to prevent infection.

Because of its mild nature, German chamomile *(Matricaria recutita)* is very useful for routine skin care. Chamomile has both anti-inflammatory and wound-healing activity that is associated with the essential oil and the water-soluble portion of the flowers. In a clinical study, an extract of chamomile was tested on patients who underwent dermabrasion to remove a tattoo. Half of the patients were given an extract of chamomile to apply to the wound, and half were given a placebo. The group using chamomile had significantly smaller healed wounds compared with those patients not using chamomile.[177] Chamomile is good for treating wounds in the mouth as well. The antibacterial activity associated with chamomile makes it useful in preventing infections.[178] Use chamomile as an infusion or as the essential oil diluted in a carrier oil. Many commercial products that contain chamomile are also available.

The herb comfrey *(Symphytum officinale)* has often been called knit-bone because of its ability to heal. This healing capacity has been documented in animal studies.[179] Use comfrey in a poultice or as an infusion on the skin. Although some people recommend that comfrey be taken internally, it has known liver toxicity and so should not be ingested in great quantity.

Calendula *(Calendula officinalis)* is another herb with a reputation for healing wounds. It possesses anti-inflammatory, antibacterial, and antiviral properties.[180] Its ability to promote healing has been well documented in both animal and human studies.[181] Calendula also has purported immunostimulant effects. It is the flowers of calendula that contain the healing properties; use calendula as an oil or liquid extract of the flowers.

Honey itself is not an herb, but it is derived from herbs. It has a long folk tradition of use on wounds to promote healing and prevent infection. Its application for these purposes is growing, especially in clinics in Third World countries, where it is often too expensive and difficult to find other wound medication. The high fructose levels in honey prevent the growth of microorganisms and provide the skin cells with the nourishment necessary for growth. Honey is both antimicrobial and promotes healing of wounds.[182] It makes a good medium for the dilution of other antibacterial herbs and oils. The quality of honey as a medicinal can vary widely, and it may be preferable to use organic honey that contains no pesticides. For wounds that have begun to show signs of infection—swelling, redness, or pus—an essential oil with antibacterial activity may be helpful. Lavender oil can be applied directly to the skin. Or dilute tea tree oil or thyme oil about 1:10 in a carrier oil such as almond oil.

When dealing with the skin, substances that are too toxic to be ingested can be considered for topical application. Antiseptics are agents that have a more general antimicrobial activity than antibiotics and sometimes can be used topically. Silver is one of these agents. It comes in many forms: silver nitrate, silver sulfadiazine, and silver-coated dressings. Silver has been shown to be useful on wounds, and especially against antibiotic-resistant bacteria.[183]

YEAST INFECTIONS/CANDIDA

Yeast infections are caused by a type of fungus called *Candida*. These are single-celled organisms, much larger than bacteria. They can cause severe itching, burning, and redness. The most common yeast infections affect the skin and mucous membranes, such as the mouth, genital area, anus, and folds of the skin. Sometimes the lesions produce a whitish, curdlike secretion. Burning and itching, which may be intense, are the first signs of yeast infection. Diagnosis is made by microscopic examination of a scraped piece of skin. Although yeasts are a normal part of the body's family of microorganisms, when there is an imbalance that allows them to overgrow, *Candida* becomes bothersome. People most likely to get yeast infections are those with an imbalance in their immune system. Such imbalances are prevalent in patients with diseases that cause immunosuppression (AIDS, for example), hospitalized patients with intravascular catheters, patients who have just had surgery, intravenous drug users, and patients receiving broad-spectrum antibiotics for another infection. One study showed that 19 percent of patients seen for vaginal yeast infections had received an antibiotic within the last month, making antibiotic use twice as frequent in patients with yeast infections as it is in control patients.[184]

A Personal Account

Every time Melanie took a course of antibiotics for a bacterial infection, she knew she would get a vaginal yeast infection. So each time she had a prescription for an antibiotic, her doctor also gave her one for a vaginal cream. Although she wasn't fond of taking two prescriptions, she also hated that painful, itchy feeling of a yeast infection. Melanie began looking for other options. The next time she received antibiotics, Melanie decided to try douching once a day with a weak goldenseal and chamomile tea and to eat yogurt once a day while on the antibiotics. This seemed to prevent a yeast infection from occurring, and she felt better about not taking two prescriptions at once.

Most women are familiar with yeast infections; an estimated 75 percent of them will get one during their lifetime.[185] It is the most common opportunistic infection in women, and often takes root during a course of treatment with antibiotics for another infection. Use of oral contraceptives, obesity, pregnancy, and diabetes also contribute to yeast infection. When *Candida* infection occurs in the mouth, it is referred to as thrush. This form of the infection is seen in immunosuppressed patients, denture wearers, people with diabetes and anemia, and those receiving antibiotics or corticosteroids for other conditions. Thrush forms white patches in the mouth and is usually painful. Although yeast infections resolve quickly, they can worsen and spread throughout the body, especially in immunosuppressed patients. Many people find that by cutting back on refined sugars, yeast infections are better controlled.

Yeast infections can be helped by keeping the area clean and dry. Denture wearers who have problems with *Candida* infections should soak the dentures in an antibacterial solution and then clean them. Berberine, a component of goldenseal *(Hydrastis canadensis)*, has demonstrated activity against *Candida*. Make a strong tea from goldenseal and use it as a mouth rinse or as a solution for soaking dentures. It can also be used as a douche.[186] Traditionally, extracts of chamomile *(Matricaria recutita)* have been used orally to treat infections of the mouth. Again, the best way is to make a strong tea to use as a mouth rinse at the first sign of an oral infection. Chamomile tea has also been used successfully as a douche for vaginal infections.[187] One study found that a purified component from garlic *(Allium sativum)*, ajoene, inhibited a wide range of fungi in addition to *Candida*.[188] Garlic can be applied topically or included in the diet. (*See* chapter 8 for more information on garlic.) Eating yogurt containing active cultures of acidophilus can also alleviate yeast infections.

Echinacea pallida as well as Siberian ginseng *(Eleutherococcus senticosus)* have been shown to increase the amount of *Candida albicans* digested by white blood cells.[189] It is usually recommended that echinacea extract be taken three times a day during an active infection. Ginseng can be ingested either daily as a tea or as a liquid extract.

Tea tree oil has documented antimicrobial properties including activity against *Candida* species. In fact, when compared to the antifungal drug commonly used for yeast infections, miconazole, tea tree oil showed stronger inhibitory activity toward many fungal strains, including *Candida*.[190] A case study reported that tea tree oil was able to cure bacterial vaginosis. The patient, diagnosed with bacterial vaginitis, refused antibacterial treatment but instead used a five-day course of 200 milligrams of tea tree oil in a vegetable-oil base in the vagina. After this treatment, an examination showed her to be free from abnormal bacteria in the vagina.[191] Tea tree oil can be used in this way or as a douche. (*See* chapter 8 for more information on tea tree oil.)

Probiotics have also exhibited success in eliminating vaginal infections. Although typically thought of for treating diarrhea, *Lactobacilli* are an important normal inhabitant of the vagina as well. Reinfecting the vagina with these organisms can improve chronic and frequent recurrences of vaginitis. Women who ingested yogurt daily for six months had fewer infections than did those not ingesting yogurt. Even using vaginal suppositories containing *Lactobacillus* has shown improvement.[192] Using a mild douche containing diluted yogurt could produce beneficial results as well. Make sure that your yogurt contains active cultures.

Chronic vaginitis has also been attributed to a diet high in refined sugar as well as to excessive stress or anxiety. Dr. Howard Smith, of New Mexico, believes that stress can lead to problems in carbohydrate metabolism and that patients with chronic vaginitis should be given help with dietary management and stress reduction.[193]

The herbalist Linda Millican suggests a warm bath containing lemon balm *(Melissa officinalis)* for sufferers of chronic yeast infection. The skin is able to absorb the healing agents of lemon balm, allowing them to be distributed throughout the body. A warm bath can also relieve some of the stress of an infection. Applying a compress of witch hazel to the vulval area also may provide relief.

8 HERBAL MONOGRAPHS

ASTRAGALUS
(Astragalus membranaceus)

Family: Leguminosae
Other names: Huang qi, milk-vetch, *Radix astragali*
Usage: Immune stimulant

GROWTH

There are more than fifteen hundred species of astragalus. These members of the Leguminosae family are used primarily as forage and ground covers. They are related to peas and indeed look very similar. *Astragalus membranaceus* will grow two to three feet tall in full sun. The roots of the plant are used for medicinal purposes and should be harvested by the fourth year of growth.

HISTORICAL USE

Astragalus membranaceus has been used as a medicinal plant in traditional Chinese medicine for thousands of years. It is considered an adaptogenic herb, or a "qi-tonifying" herb, and it is found in many

Chinese tonics. Adaptogens are used to increase overall vitality as well as to treat chronic illnesses, diabetes, and coronary heart disease. It is said to invigorate and promote tissue regeneration.

Current Use

Today many people use astragalus as an immune modulator. It can stimulate the immune system to overcome chronic infections, even cancer, or to surmount a short-term infection. It may be beneficial to take simultaneously with cancer chemotherapy to keep the immune system functioning and reduce the side effects. The herbalist Linda Millican warns not to use astragalus when the body is under severe insult or when an infection is ongoing. It is to be taken before the body becomes ill, to maintain peak performance. She suggests using the root of astragalus in stews in the fall. This will keep the body strong enough to ward off the colds and flu of winter.

Chemistry

The main medicinal components of astragalus are saponins. These are sugar-containing lipids that have soaplike characteristics. A particular polysaccharide fraction, referred to in the literature as fraction 3, named because of its size, seems to be the most active ingredient.[1] There are also a number of amino acids found in astragalus that may contribute to its activity, such as gamma-aminobutyric acid, proline, and aspartic acid, as well as polysaccharides and flavonoids. Isoflavans that have antimicrobial activity have also been identified in some astragalus species.[2]

Toxicology

There are no known adverse effects or contraindications to the use of astragalus.[3]

Pharmacology and Studies

Current studies on astragalus indicate that it is an immune modulator, antioxidant, and antiviral agent. Immune modulators, or biological-response modifiers, affect the immune system in some way to make it more active. Besides helping the body eliminate both chronic and acute infectious disease, this property can aid cancer patients. Because cancer chemotherapy typically affects the cells of the blood and depresses the immune system, cancer patients are prone to infections. A biological-response modifier can lessen the toxic side effects of chemotherapy and improve a patient's quality of life. This same immune-modulating activity stimulates the immune system to act on chronic infections to eliminate them.

The immune-stimulating effects of astragalus have been documented in laboratory studies. The addition of astragalus to a dish of white blood cells and tumor cells stimulated the white blood cells to attack the tumor cells. When combined with the immune-enhancing chemical interleukin-2, astragalus enhanced the effects of interleukin-2, allowing a lower dose to be administered.[4] Sometimes tumor cells have the ability to impair the function of white blood cells. This action can be confirmed in the laboratory by combining white blood cells with tumor cells. In one experiment, when astragalus was added to the combination of white blood cells and tumor cells, it was able to block this negative effect of the tumor cells on the white blood cells. Additional experiments have also found that astragalus has a variety of stimulatory effects on white blood cells in mice.[5, 6] Immune-stimulating effects have also been shown in immunodepressed mice. By injecting the immunosuppressive drug cyclophosphamide into mice, their immune systems can be knocked out. If these "knock-out" mice are then injected with extracts from astragalus, their immune systems are restored.[7] Unfortunately, studies are lacking in humans.

One study was conducted on patients with lung cancer. These patients were receiving the standard medical treatment of chemotherapy, radiotherapy, and immunotherapy but with the addition of a traditional Chinese medicine containing astragalus. This supplementation of standard treatment improved their overall response rate.[8] Although this study was not comparative, it does indicate that astragalus may be useful as an immune modulator in conjunction with cancer chemotherapy. Extracts from astragalus also reversed the suppression of macrophages caused by tumor cells.[9]

In animal studies, astragalus has proved useful in treating viral myocarditis. This disease is caused by the enterovirus Coxsackie B, which also infects humans, causing viral heart disease. Mice were injected with a water-soluble extract from astragalus just before being inoculated with the Coxsackie virus, to induce myocarditis. When compared with a control group that was given the virus alone, the group that received astragalus had far fewer heart lesions. When the actual amount of virus in the heart was measured, the astragalus group also had fewer viruses.[10] Another study showed that *Astragalus membranaceus* extract prevented the Coxsackie virus from reproducing.[11]

These immune-modulating effects demonstrated by astragalus indicate multiple uses for the herb, including prevention against contracting infectious disease.

CHAMOMILE
(Matricaria recutita and Chamaemelum nobile)

Family: Compositae/Asteraceae
Other names: German chamomile *(Matricaria recutita)*,
  Hungarian chamomile, sweet false chamomile, wild chamomile, manzanilla, Roman chamomile *(Chamaemelum nobile)*
Usage: Anti-inflammatory, sedative, antimicrobial, soothes
  gastrointestinal disturbances

GROWTH

There are many different plants that have been called chamomile (also spelled camomile.) The two most commonly used chamomile plants are German chamomile *(Matricaria recutita)* and Roman chamomile *(Chamaemelum nobile)*. These plants share a typical daisylike flower and a fragrant, applelike smell. In *Greek, chamomile* means "ground apple," and its name in Spanish, *manzanilla*, means "little apple." While German chamomile grows to two to three feet, Roman chamomile is low growing and is often used as a ground cover. Its leaves are fine and featherlike. Both plants flourish throughout Europe, Africa, Asia, and North America. It is the flower heads that are used medicinally.

HISTORICAL USE

Chamomile is one of the most well-known and most often used herbs. Both popular forms of chamomile have traditionally been used to treat conditions involving muscle spasms, such as indigestion and menstrual cramps. Because it is anti-inflammatory and soothing to the skin, it can be found in many skin-care products. It is also said to have sedative effects that promote sleep, relieve nightmares, decrease stress, and calm nervous afflictions and hysteria.

CURRENT USE

Its anti-inflammatory activity has made chamomile a soothing remedy for skin ailments, and it can be found in many skin-care products. Soothing chamomile tea is used as a sedative to relieve stress and promote sleep. Its gentle action makes it particularly useful for children. Other uses include as an antiseptic mouthwash, to promote digestion, and to relieve muscle spasms.

CHEMISTRY

Most of the therapeutic effects of chamomile are due to the volatile oils as well as the flavonoids found in the flower heads. The volatile oils in German chamomile include alpha-bisabolol, bisabolol oxides, and farnesene; in Roman chamomile these oils are aliphatic esters.[12] Chamazulene, found only in the essential oil and obtained by steam distillation, gives the oil its characteristic scent and blue color.[13, 14]

Chamomile also contains high-molecular-weight polysaccharides, which have been associated with immunostimulating activity. It is the family of molecules known as coumarins that is responsible for chamomile's antibacterial properties. These coumarins include umbelliferone and its methyl ester, heniarin.[15]

TOXICOLOGY

Many allergic reactions, and even a few anaphylactic reactions, have been reported with chamomile, although the specific species was not documented in most cases. It is believed that some of the allergic reactions were due to contamination of the chamomile products by other species that are more allergenic, such as dog chamomile *(Anthemis cotula)*. Allergies to chamomile are thought to cross-react with other members of the Compositae family, such as ragweed, arnica, yarrow, feverfew, tansy, and artemisia. People allergic to any of these plants should also stay away from chamomile. High doses of Roman chamomile have been reported to cause nausea and vomiting. However, chamomile is generally considered to be a very safe herb, even for children.[16, 17]

STUDIES

The German Commission E, a governmental department that evaluates herbs scientifically, approves chamomile for the treatment of bacterial infections of the skin, oral cavity, and gums.[18] Very few medical studies have been conducted using chamomile, and most of the evidence of its antimicrobial effect is based on historical and empirical data. The antibacterial properties of chamomile may be due to coumarins, which are found in both types of chamomile. Chamazulene, an ingredient occurring at somewhat higher levels in German chamomile, possesses antifungal activity. Chamomile extracts were also found to inhibit the growth of *Staphylococcus aureus*, *Candida albicans*, and *Trichonomonas vaginalis*.[19] An ethanol extract of German chamomile has been reported to inhibit both poliovirus and herpesvirus.[20] A mouthwash of chamomile can be used against mucosal infections, providing both cooling and astringent effects. Large polysaccharides from German chamomile have also been reported to have immunostimulating activity.[21]

Chamomile is perhaps most effective as an anti-inflammatory agent. This property partners well with its antimicrobial activity, as inflammation often accompanies infection. Because the antimicrobial activity of chamomile is milder than that of other herbs, it is best used in a preventive capacity. Chamomile is often applied to skin conditions such as eczema and psoriasis. These are inflammatory conditions that sometimes become infected from breaking of the skin through constant scratching. One study showed that a commercial cream containing chamomile, Kamillosan, was comparable to Fluocortin and bufexamac for relieving the inflammation associated with skin problems such as eczema.[22] For this reason, chamomile has also been used to treat diaper rash as well as skin wounds. One clinical study showed that when chamomile was combined with an antibiotic, it improved the symptoms of hemorrhagic cystitis. In this study, patients took an oral antibiotic and received a bladder instillation of chamomile extract on the first day. Afterward, they took a daily bath containing chamomile. After ten days, it was found that the group that took chamomile baths had fewer symptoms than did the group receiving antibiotic alone.[23] Chamomile can also speed up the healing of wounds. This was demonstrated in a double-blind study using chamomile extracts on the sites of dermabrasion.[24]

Echinacea
(Echinacea purpurea, E. angustifolia)

Family: Compositae/Asteraceae
Other names: Purple coneflower, Sampson root, droops
Usage: Immune stimulant

Growth

Although its common name is the purple coneflower, owing to widespread knowledge of its medicinal activity it is usually referred to by its botanical name, echinacea. There are many different species of echinacea, three of which are used medicinally: *E. purpurea, E. angustifolia,* and *E. pallida.* The *angustifolia* species was a plant native to the midwestern plains of the United States, but now its abundant use has come close to eliminating the plant from the wild. The plant, which has a beautiful purple, cone-shaped flower on a bristly stem, stands two to three feet tall. It tolerates the heat of summer without requiring lots of water and so is a welcome addition to any garden. In fact, growing it in your garden is a good idea, as its popularity is reflected by its dwindling populations in the wild.

Historical Use

Native Americans used the root of echinacea as a blood purifier. Although it is difficult to explain its effect scientifically, it was taken for many ailments, including infections, bee stings, snakebites, and rheumatism. It was from the Native Americans that the European settlers learned the value of echinacea. Very popular in the 1920s, echinacea declined in use and availability with the development of antibiotics. Its main purpose gradually became that of an immune stimulant used to treat a variety of infections, inflammations, and fever.

CURRENT USE

Interest in the use of echinacea has blossomed again. Today, echinacea is widely used as an immune stimulant to prevent or shorten the duration of colds and flu. It is also used as an antiseptic and antiviral agent and to dilate blood vessels.

CHEMISTRY

Echinacea produces many medicinal compounds, with some slight differences among species. The components most likely to stimulate the immune system are the high-molecular-weight polysaccharides, such as echinacin. Polysaccharides are long chains of small sugar molecules connected to each other. *E. purpurea* and *E. angustifolia* contain similar amides in their oil-soluble portions, whereas *E. pallida* contains polyenes in its oil-soluble portion. Differences notwithstanding, both of these compounds probably have medicinal activity.[25]

Dr. Varro Tyler says that tinctures of echinacea made from alcohol and water are most active and absorbed more readily than tablets or capsules. Keep in mind that even in tincture, echinacea quickly loses its effectiveness. If the tincture imparts a tingling sensation to the tongue, it is probably active, but the most active echinacea extracts even have a salty taste. This effect on the tongue derives from the polysaccharide echinacin in the mixture.[26]

TOXICITY

Echinacea contains pyrrolizidine alkaloids, which can be toxic to the liver but probably not in the doses used for immune-stimulating effects. These compounds are similar to the liver toxins found in comfrey.[27] Because echinacea stimulates the immune system, there is some concern that it might exacerbate such autoimmune diseases as lupus, scleroderma, multiple sclerosis, and rheumatoid arthritis.

This immune-stimulating activity could also be harmful to those undergoing immunosuppressive therapy—for example, patients who have undergone an organ transplant.[28] Very little is known about the long-term toxicity of echinacea, so it should not be taken for long periods. The herbalist Christopher Hobbs suggests using echinacea for a week to ten days. If symptoms persist, take it another week to ten days, but only after a hiatus of a few days.[29] Continued use of echinacea, in fact, can depress the immune system. Echinacea is part of the same family as ragweed—allergy sufferers should beware.

PHARMACOLOGY AND STUDIES

Although it is still favored among herbalists, clinical studies have been confusing mainly due to the many different types of echinacea extracts used, including expressed juice, alcohol extracts, and dried herb in capsules. Some studies have used injections of echinacea instead of oral doses, a form most consumers are not interested in. However, empirical evidence seems to win out in the case of echinacea and people continue to use it.

Laboratory, or in vitro studies, as well as animal studies, have produced overwhelming evidence, that echinacea can stimulate the activity of white blood cells in a variety of ways. Echinacea promotes the proliferation of white blood cells, movement of white blood cells to the site of an infection, engulfing of bacteria by white blood cells, activation of T cells, and production of interferon and interleukin.[30]

Older meta-analyses and clinical studies have come up short in providing proof that echinacea is effective in stimulating the immune system. Newer studies are beginning to give better documentation though. One recent study, which included 302 volunteers, showed that echinacea did decrease the rate of upper respiratory tract infection. However, it was only a modest 10 to 20 percent decrease.[31] Another study, which enrolled 108 patients, showed that those taking echinacea extract had fewer colds and their duration was two days shorter than for volunteers not taking echinacea.[32] Again, a rather modest improvement over control.

In this study, volunteers who had a history of frequent colds took 4 milliliters, twice a day, of alcohol-based echinacea extract for eight weeks. With increased consumer interest in echinacea, additional clinical studies will be designed so that laboratory experiments suggesting an effect on the immune system can be either confirmed or denied. Trials can also supply us with a more accurate knowledge of effective dosing and can tell us what form of echinacea extract is most effective.

Echinacea also has demonstrated antibacterial properties, as well as antiviral activity against the herpesvirus, influenza virus, and vesicular virus. A new topical treatment for herpes, called Viracea (Destiny BioMedix Corporation), contains benzalkonium chloride and extracts of *Echinacea purpurea*. This cream has been shown to be effective against many strains of herpes simplex virus 1 and 2, including strains resistant to acyclovir.[33] Additional studies have indicated that echinacea extracts improve wound healing and act as an anti-inflammatory agent. It can be used topically on eczema, psoriasis, herpes lesions, and wounds.[34]

GARLIC
(Allium sativum)

Family: Amaryllidaceae/Liliaceae
Other names: Ajo
Usage: Antimicrobial, heart tonic

GROWTH

Like the onion, to which it is related, garlic produces an underground bulb and linear leaves that arise from its base. During the summer, white to pink flowers grow on a tall stem. Although most of the garlic we eat is domesticated, it also grows wild in many places.

HISTORICAL USE

Numerous legends surround the uses of garlic, from its power to build strength and endurance to its reputation for the ability to ward off evil spirits to its addition to magical brews. It has traditionally been popular as a culinary herb and it also has had a long history of medicinal use for headache, to prevent plague, as an antidote for poisoning by hemlock and henbane, and to treat infectious diseases. It has been administered for a number of fungal diseases, such as ringworm, and for chronic bronchitis and colds. In early Greece, garlic was thought to cleanse the digestive tract. It was even taken as a diuretic and as a cure for baldness. Garlic has also been used to treat insect bites and stings.

CURRENT USE

The benefits touted for garlic are still manifold, and many have stood the test of modern science. Its most famous application is in treating heart disease. It has a number of actions that make it a useful heart medicine, among them lowering serum cholesterol and triglyceride levels, increasing the formation of high-density lipoproteins, and blocking the formation of blood clots. It allows the blood vessels to relax, thus reducing blood pressure. Garlic also possesses antimicrobial activity against bacteria, fungi, and yeasts as well as many viruses. There is evidence that garlic may protect the liver from damage caused by toxins and stimulate the immune system as well. Its use in cooking developed in southern Europe, and there are now numerous recipes that call for garlic. Recipes for garlic remedies also abound. One can find instructions for making garlic cough syrup and garlic tea as well as tinctures, oils, and vinegars.

CHEMISTRY

The chemistry of garlic is a bit complex. Garlic contains protein enzymes called allinases. These enzymes act on sulfur-containing substances found in garlic called alliin, an amino acid–like compound. Alliin is then converted to allicin as well as some minor components, such as allylpropyl disulfide. The garlic clove must be crushed for this conversion to take place. Additional medicinal components of garlic are ajoene and S-allylmercaptocysteine. These components of garlic are all volatile oils that are easily recognized by their odiferous sulfur content. Garlic preparations made by heat or solvent extraction are probably not medicinally active because of the lack of enzymes.[35]

TOXICOLOGY

No toxic effects have been reported with the widespread use of garlic in cooking. In some people, however, garlic can produce burning in the mouth or on the skin. If you are prone to this skin irritation, it may help to apply a protective layer of oil to the area first and then rub the garlic on top.[36] Alternatively, crush garlic between gauze sheets and apply that to the skin. Anyone receiving anticoagulation therapy should not use large amounts of garlic, as garlic has a similar anticoagulant effect. Very high doses of garlic, more than what would be used in food, may have serious side effects.

PHARMACOLOGY AND STUDIES

Garlic has been shown to have significant antimicrobial activity against bacteria, fungi, viruses, and protozoa. The pathogens subject to garlic's activity include *Staphylococcus, Escherichia, Proteus, Salmonella, Providencia, Citrobacter, Klebsiella, Hafnia, Aeromonas, Vibrio, Bacillus,* and *Mycobacterium tuberculosis.*[37, 38] Garlic is also active against a number of fungi that are involved in skin infections. In fact, garlic has been shown to inhibit nearly all of the organisms that cause tinea, or ringworm and athlete's foot infections, as well as yeasts (*Candida* spp.)[39, 40] A clinical study in humans found that a compound present in garlic was effective in treating athlete's foot. In this study, a cream containing 0.4 percent ajoene was used. After seven days of treatment, 79 percent of patients were free of the fungus that caused athlete's foot.[41] Raw garlic, as well as commercial preparations of garlic, were also found to have antimicrobial activity against *Helicobacter pylori,* the organism responsible for stomach ulcers in many people.[42] When comparing people with and without *H. pylori* infections, epidemiological studies found that the more garlic consumed, the lower the chance of being infected with *H. pylori.*[43] This should be enough evidence to keep garlic on hand and to use it liberally.

Effects on the immune system as well as prevention of cancer have been documented for garlic. Organosulfur compounds of garlic can augment the function of both macrophages and T-lymphocytes.[44] Aged garlic extracts have been shown to be effective against bladder cancer. Garlic extracts were injected subcutaneously into mice with bladder cancer (transitional cell carcinoma). These mice showed significant reduction in tumor growth compared to mice not receiving garlic extracts. Garlic extract was also effective when given orally. Toxicity was seen when garlic was used at high doses, but an effective therapeutic window was found with no side effects.[45]

Laboratory, epidemiological, and clinical data support the use of garlic to prevent heart disease and atherosclerosis. This is due to garlic's ability as an antithrombotic agent, a vasodilatory agent, and a lipid-lowering agent.[46] A recent meta-analysis of clinical data showed that one half to one clove of garlic per day was effective in lowering total serum cholesterol levels by about 9 percent.[47]

GOLDENSEAL
(Hydrastis canadensis)

Family: Ranunculaceae
Other names: Yellow root, ground raspberry
Usage: Infections

GROWTH

Goldenseal is native to the moist, shady woodlands of eastern North America. Although once abundant, goldenseal is close to being endangered because of overharvesting and the disappearance of habitat. Because the active part is the root, the entire plant is sacrificed. The plant is low growing and produces small white and green flowers, and orange-red berries in the fall. Its name derives from the small, seal-shaped scars found on the rhizome. Because of its scarcity in the wild, this herb would make a good addition to your herb garden if you have the right conditions: shade and moist soil.

HISTORIC USE

This herb was used by Native Americans to treat a variety of skin infections and gastrointestinal problems; European settlers used it as a dye plant. Goldenseal, as well as its constituents hydrastine and berberine, was once common ingredients in eyewashes.

CURRENT USE

Berberine has antibiotic, immunostimulant, anticonvulsant, sedative, hypotensive, uterotonic, choleretic, and carminative properties. The herb is used primarily to treat infections. Unlike echinacea, which is taken to prevent infections, berberine is administered after the advent of an infection, to fight an entrenched cold. To relieve inflammation and infection in the nose, it can be used as a snuff. Take it in powdered form or use as a salve, tincture, or tablet. The herbalist Steven Foster suggests not using goldenseal for more than two weeks at a time.[48]

CHEMISTRY

Two major alkaloids are found in goldenseal—berberine and hydrastine. Minor alkaloids include berberastine, canadine, and candaline. Purified berberine has been used by the medical establishment to treat malaria and to relieve colic, gas, and fevers. Berberine is found in other plants that have similar therapeutic activity, including Oregon grape root (*Mahonia* spp.), goldthread (*Coptis* spp.), bloodroot *(Sanguinaria canadensis)*, shrub yellow root *(Xanthorrhiza simplicissima)*, and barberry (*Berberis* spp.).

TOXICOLOGY

Because berberine and other alkaloids in goldenseal act on smooth muscle, such as that of the uterus, goldenseal should not be taken internally during pregnancy. In fact, it has been used as an abortifacient. Its effects on the heart are to stimulate it at low doses and slow it down it at higher doses. For this reason, people with heart problems should also stay away from goldenseal. Although the herb has been widely used without reports of toxic reactions and is considered to be nontoxic, very little is known about the long-term effects of goldenseal; thus, it is not recommended for use over the long term.[49] Because of its antibiotic properties, goldenseal may alter the normal bacterial environment of the intestines. This may have repercussions that include changes in nutrient absorption. After taking goldenseal, it is advisable to also take a probiotic, such as yogurt, to replace the intestinal bacteria.

stomach ulcers

PHARMACOLOGY AND STUDIES

Goldenseal and berberine are widely known as antimicrobial. Goldenseal has demonstrated activity toward a number of yeasts, bacteria, fungi, and parasites. Specific pathogens of interest include *Helicobacter pylori*, which is involved in stomach ulcers, and antibiotic-resistant *Mycobacterium tuberculosis*, which causes tuberculosis.[50, 51] It has been used for skin infections, vaginal infections, and eye infections. There is also evidence that goldenseal stimulates the immune system. One study showed that goldenseal treatment increased antibody production.[52]

Berberine has also demonstrated effectiveness against diarrhea. A single 400 milligram dose of berberine sulfate improved diarrhea symptoms due to *E. coli* or *Vibrio cholerae*.[53] Preliminary studies have also found berberine to have antitumor activity and to stimulate bile, thus aiding digestion.[54]

LEMON BALM
(Melissa officinalis)

Family: Labiatae
Other names: Balm, grapefruit mint
Usage: Antiviral, antibacterial, fights cold sores, calmative, mild sedative

GROWTH

Lemon balm was brought to the United States by early settlers, who may have used it to lift their spirits in a new land. It grows quickly and can be invasive under the right conditions. Its leaves are rather coarse, and it produces very small white, pinkish, or yellowish flowers in late summer. The plant itself reaches a height of two to three feet. Bees love lemon balm, so keep your distance.

HISTORICAL USE

Lemon balm has long been used as a medicine and as a flavoring. Part of the mint family, it has the flavor of both lemon and mint. Arabs once used lemon balm to raise their spirits and for heart disorders. It has a mild sedative effect and is a pleasant addition to tea. A Greek physician of the first century, Dioscorides, suggested lemon balm to treat the bites of insects and dogs. Old European herbals claim that using it can improve memory.

Current Use

Today we know that lemon balm has antiviral and antibacterial properties. Its common use is in skin balms and lip ointments to prevent cold sores. Many people find that lemon balm taken in tea can be calming and will relieve a headache.

Chemistry

The essential oil of lemon balm contains citral, citronellol, geraniol, limonene, linalool, and pinene. Melissa also contains phenolic and antioxidant compounds including rosmarinic acid, caffeic acid, and thymol.[55]

Toxicology

There are no known toxicities associated with lemon balm, and it is thought to be safe for long-term usage.

Pharmacology and Studies

Extracts from lemon balm are antimicrobial with antiviral activity against HIV and HSV-1, the virus that causes cold sores.[56] In Germany, lemon balm is widely used as a treatment for herpes and cold sores. Studies there have shown that a cream containing lemon balm can prevent recurrence of cold sores as well as interrupt the progression of cold sores, and also promotes healing.[57] The compound rosmarinic acid found in lemon balm has been found to have some anti-inflammatory effect in laboratory studies, but there has been no documentation of this effect in humans.[58]

LICORICE
(*Glycyrrhiza glabra* and other species)

Family: Leguminosae
Other names: Liquorice, licorish, Scythian root
Usage: Anti-inflammatory, antimicrobial, bronchitis,
   digestive problems, gastric ulcers

GROWTH

The licorice plant has a long, branching taproot that is used medicinally. The plant grows in rich, moist soils, often near river valleys, but it prefers hot, dry conditions in summer. It has delicate foliage and grows to a height of three to seven feet, producing white or purple flowers in midsummer, followed by seedpods.

HISTORICAL USE

The sweet root of licorice is best known as a flavoring, specifically for candy. Traditions in most countries recognize its medicinal qualities. It also has a history of medicinal applications as a cough remedy, as a mild laxative, to reduce water retention, for such respiratory conditions as bronchitis and congestion, and for digestive conditions, such as ulcer and colic. It has also been added to eyedrops to treat inflammation.

CURRENT USE

Today licorice is commonly taken for respiratory conditions. It can quiet a dry cough, loosen congestion in the chest, and soothe a sore throat. It may also protect the liver from damage due to toxins. Because it contains antimicrobial and antiviral compounds, it is used to fight infections. Because of its hormonal effects it is used for adrenocortical insufficiency and for stress. The drug carbenoxolone has been isolated from licorice for use as a treatment for stomach ulcers. Brewers add licorice to dark beers, such as porters and stouts.

anti-ulcer drug

CHEMISTRY

The major component of licorice is a terpenoid glycoside called glycyrrhizin. This agent contributes not just the sweet taste to licorice, but its medicinal effects and its side effects as well. Licorice contains a variety of other polyphenols that act as antioxidants, such as formononetin, glabrin, glabrol, glabrone, and glyzarin. There are many volatile oils in licorice, including anethole, benzaldehyde, eugenol, and linalool. Active polysaccharides have also been found. Licorice also contains mucilages that have soothing qualities.[59]

TOXICOLOGY

Glycyrrhizin and glycyrrhetinic acid have steroidlike effects on the body that can lead to sodium retention and potassium loss. Both can amplify the effects of cortisol by inhibiting its breakdown. Although this allows licorice to have potent anti-inflammatory activity, it also produces a condition known as hyperaldosteronism, which leads to high blood pressure and water retention or swelling. It is not known how much licorice is needed to cause such drastic effects, and it seems to affect individuals in a highly variable way. These symptoms can be reversed after withdrawal of licorice, but those people who already have cardiovascular disorders should not use licorice.[60] Periodic or low doses of licorice should not cause a problem. Licorice that has had glycyrrhizin removed, DGL, is useful for ulcers but less so for other ailments.

PHARMACOLOGY AND STUDIES

Licorice has confirmed antimicrobial activity—owing to its isoflavonoid content as well as its glycyrrizin content—against various bacteria and yeasts. These include *S. aureus* and *Candida albicans.*[61] In fact, according to the ethnobotanist Dr. James Duke, licorice contains more known antibiotic compounds than any other herb.[62]

Licorice also has antiviral activity toward a number of viruses, due to glycyrrhizin. When glycyrrhizin was given to mice infected with lethal amounts of influenza virus, it provided protection from lung damage and death.[63] In Japan, licorice is sometimes given intravenously to treat hepatitis B infections.[64] Herpesvirus is also inhibited by extracts of licorice. In fact, when glycyrrhizin was administered intraperitoneally to mice before lethal infection with HSV-1, the mice were protected and survival was significantly increased over the control group.[65] When using licorice for its antiviral activity, be sure not to use a deglycyrrhizinated product, however; it is precisely that compound that is necessary for its antiviral actions. These compounds also have a history of use in protecting the liver from damage caused by toxins or viruses. They are commonly used in China for such purposes.[66] Its antimicrobial properties are complemented by its immune-stimulating activity. A recent study showed that polysaccharides from licorice were able to stimulate macrophage activity.[67]

Also attributed to licorice is anti-inflammatory activity, which stems from its inhibitory effect on cortisol degradation.[68] Licorice also has soothing qualities that can relieve ulcer symptoms. In fact, the frequently used ulcer drug carbenoxolone is isolated from licorice.[69] This, combined with licorice's antibacterial qualities, might make it an important treatment for ulcers caused by *H. pylori*.

anti-ulcer

MYRRH
(Commiphora myrrha)

Family: Burseraceae
Other names: Mirra, *Balsamodendron myrrha*, myrrhin
Usage: Antimicrobial

GROWTH

Myrrh was one of the royal gifts from the Magi to the Christ child. No wonder this herb is so valuable. It has been used for medicine, embalming, and pain relief. Myrrh is a knotty shrub or small tree native to the deserts of northeast Africa and the Middle East. The gummy resin, which hardens to a brittle, reddish clump, is used medicinally. It has long been burned in religious ceremonies and rituals for its aroma as well. The Egyptians also used an oil containing myrrh for embalming. Myrrh can be obtained as a tincture or in the form of resin or powder made from the leaves and stem.

HISTORICAL USE

Myrrh has traditionally been used as a healing and astringent herb. It has been said to heal skin ulcers, such as bedsores, and rotting teeth or gums. It is also said to promote labor.

CURRENT USE

Although not well known, myrrh has antibacterial properties and is used to heal a variety of skin infections, such as eczema, athlete's foot, chapped skin, and gum and mouth infections, and for wounds and sores. It is also said to be good for aging skin and wrinkles.

Taken as a gargle, it may relieve a sore throat. It is often used to treat upper respiratory tract infections. Its essential oil may have decongestant properties when diluted in oil and applied to the chest.

CHEMISTRY

The oil from myrrh is high in aldehydes and phenols, the main active components being the sesquiterpenes furanoeudesma-1,3-diene and curzarene. The resin from myrrh also has medicinal constituents, primarily owing to the acids it contains, including acetate, formate, myrrholate, palmitate, and phenols.

TOXICOLOGY

Because it is not a widely used herb, toxicity data is lacking. It is best used topically. If you use it internally, use it cautiously. It should not be used during pregnancy, as it may promote labor.

PHARMACOLOGY AND STUDIES

The antiseptic and antimicrobial activity of myrrh makes it useful as a topical agent for treating wounds or as a mouth rinse. There is some evidence that myrrh relieves pain. When an extract from myrrh was administered to mice, they were able to withstand more discomfort than could mice not treated with myrrh. Myrrh affects the brain's opioid receptors, the same receptors affected by morphine and opium.[70] Because of its anti-inflammatory activity, it also works well as a mouthwash and gargle for mouth sores, includng thrush and sore throat.[71]

TEA
(Camellia sinensis)

Family: Theaceae
Other names: Green tea, black tea, oolong tea
Usage: Cancer prevention, antimicrobial, antioxidant

GROWTH

Tea is an old herb thought to have been used first in China in the twenty-eighth century B.C. Although China still produces much tea, most of our tea today comes from India. This shrub, a small, slow-growing evergreen, grows best in areas that have high humidity and warm climates, with acidic soil. From the leaves and buds, we get three different types of tea—green, black, and oolong. Black tea is made by completely fermenting the leaves before drying, green tea by simply drying or steaming the leaves, and oolong tea by partial fermentation before drying. In the United States, black tea is most common. It is thought that green tea has the most health-promoting benefits because the fermentation process may harm some of tea's constituents.

Historical Use

The Japanese and Chinese held elaborate tea ceremonies, which began as Buddhist rituals. It seems that tea was drunk strictly for its pleasant taste rather than as medicine. Besides steeping in water and drinking it as a brew, people also chewed the leaves.

Current Use

Research on the health benefits of tea has escalated in recent years. Tea has been found to have beneficial activity toward the cardiovascular system in reducing cholesterol levels, risk of stroke, and risk of heart disease. There is strong evidence that tea can also reduce the risk of certain cancers. Tea is also used to treat infectious disease and to stimulate the immune system. Its traditional uses as a stimulant and digestive aid still hold as well.

Chemistry

All three types of tea contain polyphenols, which are antioxidants that may be beneficial in preventing heart disease and cancer. In black tea, the main polyphenols are theaflavins and thearubigins. In green tea, the catechins epigallocatechin-3 gallate and epicathechin-3 gallate are the main polyphenols. Oolong tea contains a combination of these ingredients. Of course, tea also contains methylxanthines, the most abundant of which is caffeine.

Toxicology

Caffeine can cause hyperactivity, anxiety, and insomnia in some people. Excessive use of caffeine can affect blood pressure as well.

One study showed that excessive tea drinking, more than six cups per day, increased the risk of cancer.[72]

PHARMACOLOGY AND STUDIES

Tea demonstrates antibacterial activity toward several bacteria including *E. coli, Proteus vulgaris, Pseudomonas fluorescens, Salmonella,* and *Staphylococcus aureus.* It appears that green tea is somewhat more potent in this regard than black tea.[73] Catechins in green tea also have activity against the ulcer-causing bacteria *Helicobacter pylori.*[74] These same catechins inhibit growth of oral bacteria that cause plaque and dental caries.[75] Green tea benefits the digestive tract because even though it is antibacterial, it does not seem to affect the lactic acid-producing bacteria of the intestines.[76] Green tea also has activity against the virulent *E. coli* strain 0157:H7, as well as a detoxifying effect toward the toxin produced by that organism. When mice were infected with this bacterium, those receiving dietary green tea extract did not succumb to disease; those not receiving the supplement died.[77] Extracts of tea also have been shown to reverse the antibiotic resistance of some strains of bacteria.[78] A component of green tea has anti-inflammatory activity and has been shown to decrease the migration of neutrophils through a layer of endothelial cells.[79]

The polyphenols in green tea are strong antioxidants and can prevent many forms of cellular damage. Tea, especially green tea, also has been found to decrease the risk of many types of cancers.[80] Several studies have shown that moderate tea intake, one to three cups per day, can lower your cancer risk. Drinking too much tea, more than six cups daily, may have the opposite effect, however. When taken by patients receiving cancer chemotherapy, tea may provide a protective effect from the side effects of chemotherapy.[81] Liver protection is another attribute of tea. When rats were given a toxic level of 2-nitropropane, administration of green tea was able to decrease the amount of damage done to the liver.[82]

Tea consumption can also lower the risk of heart attack, and several studies demonstrate that tea can prevent atherosclerosis as well.[83] With all these benefits, afternoon tea becomes much more important than simply a social ritual!

TEA TREE OIL
(Melaleuca alternifolia)

Family: Myrtaceae
Other names: Australian tea tree, tea tree, ti tree
Usage: Antimicrobial

GROWTH

Tea tree oil is steam-distilled from the leaves and terminal branches of the tea tree, a small bush with slender leaves about three inches long and cream-colored flowers. The tree grows in swampy areas of New South Wales, Australia, and the leaves and branches are harvested from November to May. The use of tea tree oil is increasing beyond the means of producers to supply the oil. For this reason, inferior oils and oil diluted with related species can be found. The oil itself is watery, with a pale yellow color and a spicy, camphorous smell, sometimes described as similar to that of nutmeg.

HISTORICAL USE

Traditionally the tea tree leaves were used by the Bundajabung Aborigines of Australia to heal wounds. It was shown in 1925 by A. R. Penfold that the oil was more potent as an antiseptic and disinfectant than phenol. The Australian army and navy added tea tree oil to first-aid kits during World War II, to be used as a disinfectant. It was also added to machine oil to reduce the number of hand infections caused by abrasions.[84]

CURRENT USE

Today tea tree oil is still used as an antiseptic and antimicrobial agent, especially for acne, nail infections, and vaginal infections.

CHEMISTRY

The oil of tea tree is steam-distilled and contains at least ninety-seven components. The concentration of these constituents varies, depending on the chemotype of the tree. The main components are terpinen-4-ol, gamma-terpinene, 1,8-cineole (eucalyptol), pinene, cymene, and sesquiterpenes. The antimicrobial activity has been attributed to the terpinen-4-ol, but several other components also have antimicrobial activity. Skin irritation has been said to be caused by 1,8-cineole, but recent studies indicate that this may not be accurate. The Australian standard for tea tree oil calls for a minimum of 30 percent terpinen-4-ol and a minimum of 15 percent 1,8-cineol.[85]

TOXICITY

There have been many cases of contact dermatitis reported after the topical use of tea tree oil. The symptoms of contact dermatitis include redness and itching accompanied by a rash. Most of these cases are probably due to an allergic reaction to components of tea tree oil. Unfortunately, there is no way of knowing whether an individual will have an adverse reaction. To be safe, use a very small amount of tea tree oil the first time, to determine whether an allergic reaction might occur. Tea tree oil should not be taken internally. Ingestion of tea tree oil has resulted in central nervous system toxicity, including hallucinations and coma.[86] Abdominal pain and diarrhea are also documented results of the internal use of tea tree oil. Limit tea tree oil to external application on the skin, or use it as a mouthwash or vaginal rinse.

PHARMACOLOGY AND STUDIES

Tea tree oil is well suited for treatment of skin diseases because it is very soluble, easily penetrating the outer layers of skin. This means that it is readily absorbed—an important characteristic for an antiseptic. The essential oil of tea tree has been found to have in vitro activity against a wide range of pathogenic organisms, including fungi, bacteria, and yeasts. The fungi that are killed by tea tree oil include those that can give rise to ringworm, folliculitis, dandruff, athlete's foot, and toenail fungus. Tea tree oil can kill yeasts, among them species of *Candida,* which cause mouth and vaginal infections.[87] Many bacterial organisms that cause skin disease, such as impetigo, are also killed by this oil. One of these organisms is *Staphylococcus aureus,* which is a typical hospital-acquired infection. More important, tea tree oil can kill *S. aureus* bacteria that have become resistant to the most popular antibiotic administered to eliminate the infection, methicillin.[88] This makes it a good candidate for use in antibacterial soaps in hospitals.

Tea tree oil has been used to treat a variety of diseases, including burns, skin infections, colds and flu, thrush, sore throat, rashes, insect bites, vaginitis, acne, congestion, dermatitis, wounds, arthritis, cold sores, and infections. Double-blind, controlled clinical studies have established the effectiveness of tea tree oil in treating athlete's foot, acne, and toenail fungus, or onychomycosis. In testing for its effect on athlete's foot, patients with positive results on cultures for athlete's foot used a cream containing 10 percent tea tree oil twice a day for four weeks. Another group of patients used a standard antimycotic treatment, tolnaftate. A third group acted as a control, applying a cream containing no medication. Patients from both treatment groups showed significant improvement in their symptoms compared with the control group; 64 percent of the tea tree oil group and 57 percent of the tolnaftate group experienced relief. Statistically, improvement in the symptoms of scaling, inflammation, itching, and burning was found to be the same in both groups. Only 30 percent of the tea tree oil group, compared with 85 percent of the tolnaftate-treated group, were cured of the fungal infection that caused the athlete's foot after the four weeks. Statistically, the tea tree oil group was no better than the control group. The tolnaftate-treated group had minor skin irritation associated with treatment, while the tea tree oil group had no adverse effects. It is possible that a slightly higher percentage of tea tree oil would be more effective in curing athlete's foot.[89]

A 5 percent solution of tea tree oil was compared with a typical acne treatment, 5 percent benzoyl peroxide. Both treatments improved acne, with results using benzoyl peroxide slightly better than for tea tree oil. The benzoyl peroxide group also had more side effects than did the group using tea tree oil; these effects included scaling, itching, and drying of the skin. Again, a higher concentration of tea tree oil might have shown better results while still minimizing the unwanted side effects.[90]

A third clinical study showed that tea tree oil was effective in treating toenail fungus. In this trial, tea tree oil was compared with a typical antifungal treatment, clotrimazole. Patients applied either 100 percent tea tree oil or 1 percent clotrimazole to the infected toenail twice daily for six months. The outcomes of both groups were equally good, with 11 percent of the clotrimazole group and 18 percent of the tea tree oil group being cured of the fungal infection. Improvement in nail appearance was documented in 61 percent of the clotrimazole group and 60 percent of the tea tree oil group. Three months after treatment was stopped, positive effects persisted in both groups.[91]

An additional case study, involving one person, showed that a five-day course of douching with tea tree oil was effective at eliminating anaerobic vaginitis.[92] Because in vitro studies have confirmed that a broad range of pathogenic organisms are killed by tea tree oil, it is probably safe to assume that it can be used for a variety of skin infections. These diseases include ringworm, dandruff, athlete's foot, toenail fungus, thrush, acne, vaginitis, impetigo, and assorted wounds.

ESSENTIAL OILS AND AROMATHERAPY

The practice of aromatherapy refers to the aromatic use of essential oils from plants. These volatile oils can be obtained by the pressing or distillation of flowers, fruits, leaves, stems, roots, or bark. Because of their concentration, very few essential oils should be used full strength, and even fewer should be ingested. Aromatherapy is a rather new discipline. One of its first practitioners was Dr. Jean Valnet, of France, who treated soldiers wounded in World War II.

Essential oils are quite fragrant, and chemically are often referred to as aromatic compounds. Essential oils are different from fatty acids and are often alcohols, aldehydes, esters, ketones, or phenols. Because phenol is known as a strong antiseptic, many essential oils also have antimicrobial activity—sometimes stronger than that of phenol itself. Essential oils can also be used for stress reduction, to reduce inflammation, and to reduce pain.

ESSENTIAL OILS FOR REDUCING STRESS

The fragrance of essential oils can be relaxing and may reduce stress. Because stress can affect the immune system and make the body more prone to infections, aromatherapy may improve the body's resistance to infection. The following essential oils are useful for stress reduction:

Basil *(Ocimum basilicum)*
Bergamot *(Citrus bergamia)*
Chamomile, Roman *(Chamaemelum nobile)*
Geranium *(Pelargonium graveolens)*
Lavender *(Lavandula angustifolia)*
Lemon *(Citrus limonum)*
Marjoram *(Origanum majorana)*
Melissa or lemon balm *(Melissa officinalis)*
Rose otto *(Rosa damascena)*
Sandalwood *(Santalum album)*
Ylang-ylang *(Canangium odorata)*

When choosing essential oils, make sure that they are actually distilled from the plant rather than a synthetic replica of only one of the components of the true essential oil. Ask question of the manufacturer. Each essential oil can contain more than three hundred different types of chemicals; trying to attribute responsibility for activity to one type alone is futile. The cost of essential oils varies greatly among different types. Lemon oil is one of the least expensive and rose oil is among the most expensive. Don't be discouraged, though; even the less expensive lemon oil (at less than five dollars for 1/2 ounce) is a potent antimicrobial and can be used for a number of infections.

Aromatherapy in the form of massage is finding its way into health-care settings. Because many medical complaints are a result of stress, massage with an aromatic oil may provide great relief and could be a good form of preventive medicine.

Keep in mind, though, that essential oils can be toxic. They are best applied externally, and one needs to be particularly careful about use during pregnancy. To be safe, consult a good aromatherapy book or practitioner before using oils.[93] Oils that the aromatherapist Susan Wormwood says should not be used by anyone include bitter almond, boldo leaf, calamus, yellow camphor, horseradish, jaborandi leaf, mugwort, mustard, pennyroyal, rue, sassafras, savin, southernwood, tansy, thuja, wintergreen, wormseed, and wormwood.[94] Some individuals may have skin sensitivities or allergies to certain oils. If a reaction develops, discontinue use immediately.

THERAPEUTIC USES OF ESSENTIAL OILS

Medical research into specific uses of essential oils is in the early stages. One study found that several essential oils—tea tree oil, oregano, cinnamon leaf, aniseed, and red thyme—were toxic to head lice.[95] The same study showed that neither rosemary oil nor pine oil was effective. Although these studies have not been extended to humans, the treatment poses no harm, and there is no reason not to use these oils.

Candida, or yeast, infections have become commonplace and are difficult to treat. Essential oils that have proven effectiveness against yeast include poplar *(Populus candicans)*, thyme *(Thymus vulgaris)*, rosemary *(Rosmarinus officinalis)*, and tea tree oil *(Melaleuca alternifolia)*.[96] There are many additional essential oils that have antiseptic properties. Although they all can be used to kill unwanted bacteria on an inanimate surface, such as your countertop, they do not all act the same way on individuals. Moreover, each person has a preference for certain vapors and is intolerant of other aromas. For this reason, you must find the oil that works best for you. In one person, lavender might be the oil of choice for a given bacterium; in another person, it might be thyme.

Many people are confused as to how to use essential oils. There are almost endless ways. For a cold or sinusitis, try rimming the nostrils several times a day with a few drops of lemon oil diluted in water. Owing to the chemical composition of essential oils, much is absorbed through the skin, sometimes within twenty minutes. For this reason, they are especially good for skin infections, because they can penetrate to the underlying layers of skin. Therapeutically, you can use essential oils in all of the following applications:

- Compress
- Dry or steam inhalation (diffuser)
- Gargle
- In the bath
- Massage or skin oil
- Mister bottle

Lisa Beaubein, a massage therapist, frequently uses essential oils to treat various illnesses, as they are rapidly absorbed during a massage. For instance, Lisa will commonly use rosemary and eucalyptus oils to treat patients with the flu. She adds three drops of essential oil of rosemary and three drops of essential oil of eucalyptus to one-half ounce of carrier oil, usually almond oil. This blend eases many of the symptoms of flu and speeds recovery. The eucalyptus oil can also boost the immune system. Undiluted tea tree oil applied to pimples also yields great results. Lisa says that the oil helps bring them to a head and then dries them up. She stresses that one should not use too much essential oil though—more is not better.

Essential oils can also be diluted in a carrier oil and used as a moisturizer after a bath or shower. Dilute six to twelve drops per one-half ounce of carrier oil. A carrier oil is typically sesame, olive, apricot, almond, walnut, or grapeseed oil. Some people find the smell of olive unpleasant. Walnut oil has a high concentration of vitamin E, a good antioxidant. A few drops of an essential oil can be added straight to the bath, or blended with an equal mixture of baking soda and sea salts, or even rubbed on the skin before a bath or shower.

Inhalation of essential oils is a good treatment for colds and bronchitis. Put a few drops into hot water to let the vapors diffuse into the air. Many commercial diffusers are available for this purpose. For chest congestion, dilute essential oil of eucalyptus in a mixture of oil with beeswax added to make it a solid (*see* chapter 9 for recipe). Rub this mixture on the chest. Of course, the oils can be inhaled directly from the bottle as well, or applied to a cotton ball and kept in a ziplock bag to serve as an inhaler.

Essential Oils for Safer Insect Repellents

Did you ever use one of those bug zappers at a picnic to keep those pesky insects at bay? If so, you could have spread a mist of bacteria and viruses. Preliminary studies from Kansas State University show that as houseflies are vaporized by electric current, bacteria and virus from their bodies travel as far as six feet away. Although there is no evidence that this represents a health hazard, it might be better to try some insect-repellent herbs instead. These herbs include tansy, artemisia (mugwort), pennyroyal, peppermint, and rue. Use them to make dried flower arrangements or decorative bags filled with dried herbs to set about the table. For extra protection, add a few drops of essential oil of bergamot, chamomile, clove, eucalyptus, lavender, lemon, peppermint, or thyme. You can also add a few drops of essential oil to a carrier oil to apply to the skin as an insect repellent.

ESSENTIAL OILS AS DISINFECTANTS

To kill airborne bacteria or viruses, add a few drops of essential oil to a mister bottle of water or a water/alcohol mixture. Jean Valnet, the author of *The Practice of Aromatherapy*, believes that using essential oils in aerosol form—particularly lemon oil—should be common practice in sickrooms and hospitals. Valnet says,

> The essence of lemon is second to none in its antiseptic and bactericidal properties. The works of Morel and Rochaix have demonstrated that the vapours of lemon essence neutralise the meningococcus in 15 minutes, the typhus bacillus in less than an hour, pneumococcus in 1–3 hours, *Staphylococcus aureus* in 2 hours, and

> haemolytic streptococcus in 3–12 hours. The essence it-
> self neutralises the typhus bacillus and staphylococcus
> in 5 minutes and the diphtheric bacillus in 20 minutes.
> A few drops of lemon essence will rid an oyster of 92%
> of its micro-organisms in 15 minutes.[97]

You can spray the air or directly spray contaminated surfaces, such as doorknobs and faucets. Consider cleaning with lemon oil diluted in water: Not only will it help dissolve dirt, but it will kill germs at the same time. Added to vinegar, essential oils make a good skin toner as well as useful household cleaning products.

Essential oils are also used in food manufacturing as a preservative. This practice may have started with the age-old tradition of using ample amounts of sage in poultry dressing. Not only did sage provide flavor to the dressing, but the antimicrobial agents in the sage also killed the bacteria that are plentiful in the chicken cavity. A recent report finds that the oils of bay, cinnamon, clove, and thyme were inhibitory against a number of food-borne pathogens.[98] Incorporation of these oils into food processing may prevent some forms of food poisoning.

The following essential oils have antimicrobial properties:

Bergamot *(Citrus aurantium* spp. *bergamia)*
Cedarwood *(Cedrus atlantica)*
Chamomile, German *(Matricaria recutita)*
Chamomile, Roman *(Chamaemelum nobile)*
Cinnamon *(Cinnamomum zeylanicum)*
Clove *(Syzygium aromaticum)*
Eucalyptus (*Eucalyptus globulus* and other species)
Frankincense *(Boswellia carterii)*
Garlic *(Allium sativum)*
Geranium *(Pelargonium* spp.)
Grapefruit *(Citrus paradisi)*
Hyssop *(Hyssopus officinalis)*
Juniper *(Juniperus communis)*
Lavender (*Lavandula angustifolia, L. officinalis,* and others)
Lemon *(Citrus limonum)*

Lemon balm *(Melissa officinalis)*
Lemongrass *(Cymbopogon flexuosus)*
Manuka *(Leptospermum scoparium)*
Marigold *(Tagetes glandulifera)*
Marjoram *(Origanum majorana)*
Myrrh *(Commiphora myrrha)*
Niaouli *(Melaleuca viridiflora)*
Oregano *(Origanum vulgare)*
Ormenis flower *(Ormenis multicaulis; Chamomile maroc)*
Palmarosa *(Cymbopogon martini)*
Patchouli *(Pogostemon cablin)*
Peppermint *(Mentha piperita)*
Pine *(Pinus sylvestris)*
Ravensara *(Ravensara aromatica)*
Rosemary *(Rosmarinus officinalis)*
Sage *(Salvia officinalis)*
Sandalwood *(Santalum album)*
Spikenard *(Nardostachys jatamansi)*
Tea tree *(Melaleuca alternifolia)*
Thyme *(Thymus vulgaris)*
Yuzu *(Citrus junos)*

9 MAKING HERBAL REMEDIES

GROWING, PURCHASING, AND COLLECTING HERBS

I get my herbs from my garden. Herb gardening is the easiest type of gardening. You not only have a source for just about whatever herb you want, but you also have a sanctuary where you can go to enjoy the beauty of your plants, to relax, or to meditate. When you are with herbs daily in a garden, you develop a relationship with them and learn more about them. Most herbs are easy to grow, but first find out which ones are suited for your area. An herb that grows best in the arid West will not necessarily grow well in the humid East. Growing your own herbs also guarantees their quality and purity. Herbs can also be bought in bulk from most health food stores. They are relatively cheap in this form, but you are relying on someone else to assure you that the herbs are pure, uncontaminated, and picked at their peak. Make sure you find a dealer you can trust. For other sources, look in the back of herb magazines for mail-order possibilities.

You can also harvest your herbs from the wild. This is called wildcrafting. The best way is to find a landowner and ask permission to collect from his or her property. It is wise to collect herbs from a site that is about to undergo construction or development, as those herbs would otherwise be destroyed. Another way is to gather herbs from public property, such as national forests, in which case you must first get a permit. There are ethical issues surrounding this practice, however, and many herbs are being overcollected to the point of endangerment. If you gather herbs from the wild, please leave plenty for the next person, and make sure your identification skills are faultless.

DRYING HERBS

Be sure you can identify various herbs, and know which parts of the herb you want. Usually it is the leaf, but sometimes it is the flower or root. Pick the freshest, newest growth of leaves and flowering tops. Pick early in the day, before the hot sun has a chance to cause the oils to evaporate. When you have gathered a small bunch, wrap a rubber band around the stems and find a place where you can hang the bunch upside down. This should be a cool, dry place out of direct sunlight. The length of time it takes to dry depends on the humidity in your area. When the herbs are dry, crush them into a jar, label it, and store away from light.

MAKING HERBAL PREPARATIONS

Dried herbs can be used in a number of preparations.

TEA

An herb tea is made by pouring very hot (just less than boiling) water over herbs and steeping for about five minutes. Usually one cup of water to one or two teaspoons of herb is used. Alternatively, put the tea in a closed glass jar and place it in the sun for four to six hours. Keep the herb in a tea bag, a tea ball, or a strainer, or put the herbs in the pot and strain them from the finished tea. You may want to use distilled or charcoal-filtered water. Bottled mineral or spring water can often contain a large amount of salts or minerals that may interfere with the herbs' action. Drink the brew or use it freely to wash the body.

INFUSION

An infusion is similar to a tea, but typically stronger. To make an infusion, pour boiling water over the herb, cover it, and let it stand for fifteen to thirty minutes. Contain the herb in a tea bag, tea ball, or strainer, or filter out the herb after the infusion is made. At times it may be preferable to use a cold rather than a hot infusion. Take infusions orally, use to wash the skin, or put them into the bath.

DECOCTION

A decoction is also similar to a tea, but it is made from the woody or hard parts of the herb. Because it is more difficult to extract the beneficial components from woody material, a decoction must actually be cooked. Place the roots, barks, twigs, or chips of wood in a pot with water and simmer for ten to thirty minutes. Strain the liquid from the herbs. A decoction can be saved in the refrigerator for up to three days. Use one to two teaspoons of plant material per cup of water. Take decoctions orally, use to wash the skin, or add to the bath.

TINCTURE

A tincture extracts the water-soluble portion of the herb into alcohol. The alcohol keeps the solution from spoiling, so a tincture can last several months. To make a tincture, put about four ounces of dried, crushed herb in a jar of about two and a half cups of alcohol. The alcohol can be brandy or vodka, but it must be at least 60 proof to prevent molds from growing. Pure grain alcohol is preferred. Rubbing alcohol is poisonous taken internally—do not use it unless you are making a mixture to be applied only externally. Shake the mixture daily for two weeks, and keep it in a warm place. Strain the tincture through cloth to remove the herbs and store your tincture in a dark glass bottle in a cool place. Because tinctures are more concentrated than teas, a normal dosage is only about one dropperful.

VINEGARS

Herbs extracted in vinegars are good to use on the skin. To make a vinegar, mix about one-half cup of dried herbs with one and a half cups of cider vinegar. Let the mixture set in a warm place for two to three weeks, shaking frequently. Strain the herbs from the vinegar and store the liquid in a clean bottle. When ready to use, dilute the vinegar with six parts of clean, distilled water, then use on the face or feet or in the bath.

COMPRESSES

Compresses are a way of applying an herb to the skin. First make a decoction or an infusion. Then soak a washcloth or linen cloth in the extract and apply it to the affected skin. Compresses can be hot or cold. To increase the value of a compress, cover with plastic the area covered by cloth to encourage the herb extract to soak into the skin. Compresses can sometimes be combined with witch hazel.

POULTICES

A poultice is similar to a compress, except that the whole plant is used, not just a water extract. To make a poultice, mash the desired part of the herb in a little boiling water. When this mixture is cool enough, apply the mashed plant directly to the skin and hold in place with a gauze bandage. You can also make a poultice with ground herbs by stirring them into boiling water to make a paste. Apply the paste to the skin and hold in place with a bandage.

BATHS

It is a good idea to use herbs in a bath, as many of the constituents are absorbed through the skin and into the body. Use whatever combination of herbs you'd like by putting one-fourth to one-half cup of herbs in a muslin bag and letting the water run over the bag. You can use the bag itself in the bath to wash the skin. Besides the therapeutic quality of the herbs you choose, the warm water itself is healing, especially in terms of alleviating stress.

INFUSED OILS

An infused oil contains the oil-soluble portion of the herb. It is made by adding a large handful of crushed herb, or as much as will fit, to a cup of carrier oil. The carrier oil can be almond, apricot, grapeseed, olive, walnut, sesame, or corn. Each has its own scent and properties. I prefer almond oil, because it is easily absorbed and slow to become rancid. Do not put in more herb than can be completely covered; it can become moldy if the oil does not cover it completely. Let this mixture steep at room temperature for one to two weeks in a warm spot, shaking daily. A quicker way to make an infusion is to heat the oil slightly and add the herbs, allowing them to steep for several hours in the hot oil. With either method, strain the herbs from the oil and bottle the liquid. An infused oil can be used directly on the skin or as a balm or salve. By adding a teaspoon of vitamin E, you extend the life of the oil: vitamin E acts as an antioxidant that helps keep oil from turning rancid. The vitamin E is good for your skin as well.

RECIPES

CALENDULA-INFUSED OIL

Extracts from the flowers of calendula *(Calendula officinalis)* are known to promote healing of the skin. An infused oil of calendula can be used either directly on the skin or combined with beeswax. Make the oil as described previously, by covering a half cup of dried calendula flowers with a cup of almond oil. Steep for two weeks, strain; and add vitamin E. You can also add a few drops of essential oil of rosemary.

HEALING CALENDULA BALM

Use this balm as an ointment to apply to scrapes. It will aid healing and prevent infection. It is especially good for dry, chapped hands.

    1 ounce beeswax
    2 cups calendula-infused oil
    1 tablespoon vitamin E or 6 drops rosemary essential oil

Heat the beeswax in a saucepan until just melted. Add the calendula-infused oil and stir until combined. Remove from the stove and add the vitamin E and/or essential oil of rosemary. You can also add a few drops of any appropriate essential oil to contribute its healing properties or aromatic quality. Pour the salve into small jars and cap. If you are not going to use some right away, store in the refrigerator.

DECONGESTANT SALVE

Use this salve for colds and flu. Applied to the chest, it can relieve lung and bronchial congestion.

> ½ ounce beeswax
> 1 cup corn oil
> 6 drops eucalyptus essential oil
> 3 drops rosemary essential oil

Heat the beeswax in a saucepan until just melted. Add the oil and stir until combined. Remove from the stove and add the essential oils. Pour the salve into small jars and cap. If you are not going to use some right away, store in the refrigerator.

LIP BALM

This lip balm contains lemon balm, which can prevent cold sores when used continually. It contains more beeswax than do the other salves, making it slightly more solid for application.

> 1 ounce beeswax
> 1 cup lemon balm–infused oil
> ½ tablespoon vitamin E oil

Heat the beeswax in a saucepan until just melted. Add the oil and stir until combined. Remove from the stove and add the vitamin E. Pour the salve into small jars and cap. If you are not going to use some right away, store in the refrigerator.

ACHY MUSCLES BATH BAG

This bath bag contains herbs that are soothing for colds and flu. It is ideal for relieving congestion and muscle aches and pains. Use it for a long hot bath.

$\frac{1}{2}$ cup dried sage
$\frac{1}{2}$ cup dried marjoram
$\frac{1}{2}$ cup dried lavender
$\frac{1}{2}$ cup dried mint

Mix the herbs together and put them in a muslin bag. Place the bag under a faucet of running warm water in the bathtub. The bag can also be used as a washcloth on the skin. Smell the bag frequently to gain the full benefit of the herbs.

TEA TREE BALM

This balm contains tea tree oil, which can be used on such fungal infections as athlete's foot and infected toenails.

$\frac{1}{4}$ ounce beeswax
$\frac{1}{4}$ cup corn oil
1 teaspoon essential oil of tea tree

Heat the beeswax in a saucepan until just melted. Add the corn oil and stir until combined. Remove from the stove and add the essential oil. Pour the salve into small jars and cap. If you are not going to use some right away, store in the refrigerator.

ANTISEPTIC DEODORANT POWDER

This can be used as a general dusting powder, but it is especially useful for body odor, jock itch, and itchy feet caused by athlete's foot. Both rosemary and sage have antiseptic properties and a pleasant smell. Sage can also help reduce perspiration.

$\frac{1}{2}$ cup baking soda
$\frac{1}{2}$ cup cornstarch
1 tablespoon powdered rosemary
1 tablespoon powdered sage leaves

Mix together all ingredients with a spoon and put into a jar with holes in the lid. Use liberally under the arms or other areas of the body.

FACIAL VINEGAR FOR OILY SKIN

1/2 cup dried yarrow flowers, sage leaves, or rosemary leaves
  (or a combination)
1 1/2 cups cider vinegar

Place ingredients together in a jar, cover, and let set 2–3 weeks, shaking frequently. Strain the herbs from the vinegar and store the liquid in a clean bottle. Dilute with 6 parts of clean distilled or spring water before using. To treat acne, try adding a few drops of tea tree oil.

FACIAL VINEGAR FOR DRY SKIN

1/2 cup dried fennel leaves, rose petals, or lady's mantle leaves
  (or a combination)
1 1/2 cups cider vinegar

Place ingredients together in a jar, cover, and let set 2–3 weeks, shaking frequently. Strain the herbs from vinegar and store the liquid in a clean bottle. Dilute with 6 parts of clean distilled or spring water before using.

OTITIS

Use a couple of drops placed in the ear to relieve the pain of an earache.

1 clove garlic, smashed
1 tablespoon dried mullein flower
1/4 cup olive oil

In a small saucepan, heat all ingredients gently for 15 minutes. Let cool. Using a dropper, place a few drops into the ear canal.

THYME SYRUP

This strong-flavored but sweetened syrup is good for colds and flu. Use as is, or add some to a cup of hot herb tea. To make a cough syrup, substitute violet flowers or white horehound leaves for the dried thyme.

2 tablespoons or more dried thyme leaves
$1/4$ cup honey
$1/4$ cup water

In a saucepan, heat for 15 minutes on medium, then let stand for 30 minutes. Strain the herbs from the liquid. Store the syrup in ice-cube trays in the freezer and use as needed.

LAVENDER LEMONADE

This flavored lemonade is relaxing and enjoyable on hot afternoons.

1 12-ounce container frozen lemonade concentrate
$1/2$ cup lavender leaves and flowers
6 $1/2$ cups boiling water

Make lavender tea by pouring the boiling water over the leaves and flowers. Let steep for about 5 minutes. Strain the tea, let it cool, and mix with the lemonade concentrate. The amount of lavender can be adjusted to suit your taste.

NOTES

Chapter 1

1. Helena Curtis, *Biology* (New York, N.Y.: Worth Publishers, Inc., 1980), 333–349.
2. Thomas D. Brock, *Biology of Microorganisms* (Englewood Cliffs, N.J.: Prentice Hall, Inc., 1979), 1–7.
3. Ibid., 7–11.
4. The Nobel Foundation, biographies, www.nobel.se/laureates/medicine-1908-1-bio.html
5. Kenneth F. Kiple, "The History of Disease," in Roy Porter, ed., *Medicine* (New York, N.Y.: Cambridge University Press, 1996), 16–51.
6. Ibid.
7. Ibid.
8. Ibid.
9. A. Basu, P. Garg, and S. Datta, "Vibrio cholera 0139 in Calcutta, 1992–1998," *Emerging Infectious Disease* 6 (2000): www.medscape.com.
10. Denise Mann, "Infectious Disease Modality More than Doubled," *Medical Tribune,* 8 February 1996, www.medscape.com.
11. B. E. Zimmerman and D.J. Zimmerman, *Killer Germs: Microbes and Diseases that Threaten Humanity* (Lincolnwood, Ill.: Contemporary Books, 1996), 70.
12. Ibid., 63–88.
13. Ibid.
14. G. F. Brooks, J. S. Butel, and S. A. Morse, eds., *Medical Microbiology* (Stamford, Conn.: Appleton and Lange, 1998), 700–702.
15. Ibid., 447–451.
16. Zimmerman and Zimmerman, *Killer Germs,* 166–169.
17. Brooks, Butel, and Morse, eds., *Medical Microbiology,* 499–505.
18. Ibid., 700–702.
19. F. G. Hayden, R. L. Atmar, M. Schilling, et al., "Use of the Selective Oral Neuraminidase Inhibitor Oseltamivir to Prevent Influenza," *New England Journal of Medicine,* 341 (1999): 1336.
20. P. A. Patriarca and R. A. Strikas, "Influenza vaccine for healthy adults?" *New England Journal of Medicine* 333 (1995): 933.
21. L. W. Winik, "Before the Next Epidemic Strikes," *Parade Magazine* (Feb 8, 1998): 6–9.
22. Zimmerman and Zimmerman, *Killer Germs,* 166–169.

23. Ibid., 90–98.

24. Ibid.,101–102.

25. L. M. Tierney, S.J. McPhee, M. A. Papadakis, *Current Medical Diagnosis and Treatment* (Stamford Conn.: Appleton and Lange, 1998), 1269.

26. Zimmerman and Zimmerman, *Killer Germs,* 103–109.

27. Brooks, Butel, and Morse, eds., *Medical Microbiology,* 273–275.

28. Zimmerman and Zimmerman, *Killer Germs,* 137–140.

29. Brooks, Butel, and Morse, eds., *Medical Microbiology,* 490–491.

30. Zimmerman and Zimmerman, *Killer Germs,* 140–141.

31. Brooks, Butel, and Morse, eds., *Medical Microbiology,* 488–489.

32. Zimmerman and Zimmerman, *Killer Germs,* 142–145.

33. Centers for Disease Control, HIV/AIDS Surveillance Report. www.cdc.gov/hiv/stats/hasrlink.htm

34. C. A. Thomas, K. B. Mullis, and P. E. Johnson, "What Causes AIDS? It's an Open Question," *Reason* (June 1994): 18–23.

35. Peter Duesberg, *Inventing the AIDS Virus* (Washington, D.C.: Regnery Publishing, 1996).

36. C. Farber, "Does HIV cause AIDS?" *Mothering* (Sept/Oct, 1998), 56.

37. Brooks, Butel, and Morse, eds., *Medical Microbiology,* 177–183.

38. Ibid.

39. G. T. Macfarlane and J. H. Cummings, "Probiotics and Prebotics: Can Regulating the Activities of Intestinal Bacteria Benefit Health?" *British Medical Journal* 318 (1999): 999–1003.

40. Brooks, Butel, and Morse, eds., *Medical Microbiology,* 177–183.

41. Ibid.

CHAPTER 2

1. G. J. Tortora and S. R. Grabowski, *Principles of Anatomy and Physiology,* 8th ed. (New York: HarperCollins, 1996).

2. D. D. Chiras, *Human Biology: Health, Homeostasis, and the Environment,* (Saint Paul, Minn.: West Publishing Company, 1995).

3. The Nobel Foundation, biographies, www.nobel.se/laureates/medicine-1908-1-bio.html

4. Brooks, Butel, and Morse, eds., *Medical Microbiology,* 110–133.

CHAPTER 3

1. American Academy of Pediatrics. www.aap.org

2. National Vaccine Information Center, 512 West Maple Avenue, Suite 206, Vienna VA 22180. www.909shot.com/

3. Ibid.

4. Ibid.

5. B. F. Elswood and R. B. Stricker, "Polio Vaccines and the Origin of AIDS," *Medical Hypothesis* 42 (1994): 347–354.

6. Randall Neustaedter, *The Vaccine Guide* (Berkeley, Calif.: North Atlantic Books, 1996), 152–154.

7. A. Rock, "Special Report/Your Health," *Money* 25 (1996): 148–161.

8. The Association of American Physicians and Surgeons. www.aapsonline.org
9. A. Rock, "Special Report/Your Health," 148–161.
10. J. Weiner, J. P. Quinn, P. A. Bradford, R. V. Goering, et al., "Multiple Antibiotic-resistant *Klebsiella* and *Escherichia coli* in Nursing Homes," *Journal of the American Medical Association* 281 (1999): 517–523.
11. T.L. Smith, M. L. Pearson, K. R. Wilcox, et al., "Emergence of Vancomycin Resistance in *Staphylococcus aureus*," *New England Journal of Medicine* 340 (1999): 493–501.
12. M. P. Dore, et al., "Demonstration of Unexpected Antibiotic Resistance of Genotypically Identical *H. pylori* Isolates," *Clinical Infectious Diseases* 27 (1998): 84–89; A. A. van Zwet, C. M. J. Vandenbrouke-Grauls, J. C. Thijs, et al., "Stable Amoxicillin Resistance in *Helicobacter pylori*," *Lancet* 352 (1998): 1595.
13. K. Gupta, D. Scholes, and W. E. Stamm. "Increasing Prevalence of Antimicrobial Resistance among Uropathogens Causing Acute Uncomplicated Cystitis in Women," *Journal of the American Medical Association* 281 (1999): 736.
14. E. E. Wang, J. D. Kellner, and S. Arnold, "Antibiotic-resistant *Streptococcus pneumoniae:* Implications for Medical Practice," *Canadian Family Physician* 44 (1998): 1881–1888.
15. J. Davies, "Bacteria on the Rampage," *Science* 383 (1996): 219–220.
16. G. G. Khachatourians, "Agricultural Use of Antibiotics and the Evolution and Transfer of Antibiotic-resistant Bacteria," *Canadian Medical Association Journal* 159 (1998): 1129–1136.
17. M. S. Al-Ghamdi, F. El-Morsy, Z. H. Al-Mustafa, et al., "Antibiotic Resistance of *Escherichia coli* Isolated from Poultry Workers, Patients and Chicken in the Eastern Province of Saudi Arabia," *Tropical Medicine and International Health* 4 (1999): 278–283.
18. K. E. Smith, J. M. Besser, C. W. Hedberg, et al., "Quinolone-resistant *Campylobacter jejuni* Infections in Minnesota, 1992–1998," *New England Journal of Medicine* 340 (1999): 1525–1532.
19. Khachatourians, "Agricultural Use of Antibiotics," 1129–1136.
20. E. Jawetz, "Penicillins and Cephalosporins," in *Basic and Clinical Pharmacology*, ed. Bertram G. Katzung (Appleton and Lange, Norwalk, Conn., 1995), 680–692.
21. E. Jawetz, "Chloramphenicol and Tetracylcines," in *Basic and Clinical Pharmacology*, 693-698.
22. Ibid.
23. F. A. Waldvogel, "New Resistance in Staphylococcus aureus," *The New England Journal of Medicine* 340 (1999): 556-557.
24. E. Jawetz, "Antifungal Agents," in *Basic and Clinical Pharmacology*, 723–729.
25. D. B. Robertson and H. I. Maibach, "Dermatologic Pharmacology," in *Basic and Clinical Pharmacology*, 932–948.
26. Ibid.
27. I. M. Kageyama, S. Sato, H. Kamiyama, et al., "Emergence of Resistance to Acyclovir and Pencyclovir in *Varicella-zoster* Virus and Genetic Analysis of Acyclovir-resistant Variants," *Antiviral Research* 40 (1999): 155–166.

28. E. E. Jawetz, "Antiviral Chemotherapy and Prophylaxis," in *Basic and Clinical Pharmacology,* 730-737.

29. Hayden, Atmar, Schilling, et al., "Use of the Selective Oral Neuraminidase Inhibitor Oseltamivir to Prevent Influenza," 1336.

30. Jean Valnet, *The Practice of Aromatherapy* (Rochester, Vt.: Healing Arts Press, 1990).

CHAPTER 4

1. B. Bower, "Stress Hormone May Speed Up Brain Aging," *Science News* 153 (1998): 263.

2. R. Glaser, B. Rabin, and M. Chesney, "Stress-induced Immunomodulation, Implications for Infectious Diseases," *Journal of the American Medical Association* 281 (1999): 2268.

3. S. W. Key, D. J. DeNoon, and S. Boyles, "Stress Speeds Progression to AIDS," *AIDS Weekly Plus* (24 May, 1999): 6–8.

4. R. Glaser, J. K. Kiecolt-Glaser, W. B. Malarkey, et al., "The Influence of Psychological Stress on the Immune Response to Vaccines," *Annals of the New York Academy of Sciences* 840 (1998): 649–655.

5. C. Wu, "Vitamin C Lowers Stress Hormone in Rats," *Science News* 156 (1999): 158.

6. Steven Foster, "Stress Less," *Herbs for Health* (May/June 1999): 38–42.

7. David Hoffman, *The Herbal Handbook: A User's Guide to Medical Herbalism* (Rochester, Vt.: Healing Arts Press, 1988), 180.

8. Carol A. Newall, Linda A. Anderson, and J. David Phillipson, *Herbal Medicines: A Guide for Health-Care Professionals* (London: The Pharmaceutical Press, 1996), 183–186.

9. Ibid., 141–150.

10. Ibid.

11. Michael A. Weiner and Janet A. Weiner, *Herbs That Heal* (Mill Valley, Calif.: Quantum Books, 1994), 292–293.

12. S. Sinclair, "Chinese Herbs: A Clinical Review of *Astragalus, Ligusticum,* and *Schizandrae,*" *Alternative Medicine Review* 3 (1998): 338–343.

13. T. Fujihashi, H. Hara, T. Sakata, et al., "Anti Human Immunodeficiency Virus (HIV) Activities of Halogenated Gomisin J Derivatives, New Nonnucleoside Inhibitors of HIV Type 1 Reverse Transcriptase," *Antimicrobial Agents and Chemotherapy* 39 (1995): 2000–2005.

14. Weiner and Weiner, *Herbs That Heal,* 70–72.

15. J. N. Dhuley, "Therapeutic Efficacy of Ashwagandha Against Experimental Aspergillosis in Mice," *Immunopharmacology and Immunotoxicology* 20 (1998): 191–198.

16. Weiner and Weiner, *Herbs That Heal,* 277–278.

17. Ibid., 174–176.

18. T. K. Chatterjee, A. Chakrabarty, M. Pathak, et al., "Effects of Plant Extract *Centella asiatica* (Linn) on Cold Restraint Stress Ulcer in Rats," *Indian Journal of Experimental Biology* 30 (1992): 889–891.

19. Susan Wormwood, *Essential Aromatherapy* (San Rafael, Calif.: New World Library, 1995).

20. K. Yamada, Y. Mimaki, and Y. Sashida, "Anticonvulsive Effects of Inhaling Lavender Oil Vapour," *Biological Pharmaceutical Bulletin* 17 (1994): 359–360.
21. K. Sembulingam, P. Sembulingam, and A. Namasivayam, "Effect of *Ocimum sanctum* (Linn) on Noise Induced Changes in Plasma Corticosterone Level," *Indian Journal of Physiology and Pharmacology* 41 (1997): 139–143.
22. Christopher Hobbs, *Stress and Natural Healing: Herbal Medicine and Natural Therapies for Depression, Anxiety, Insomnia, Heart Disease, and More* (Loveland, Colo.: Interweave Press/Botanica, 1997), 181–182.
23. Weiner and Weiner, *Herbs That Heal,* 106–107.
24. Newall, Anderson, and Phillipson, *Herbal Medicines,* 69–73.
25. N. Heneka, *"Chamomilla recutita,"* *Australian Journal of Medical Herbalism* 5 (1993): 33–39.
26. A. H. Wong, M. Smith, and H. Boon, "Herbal Remedies in Psychiatric Practice," *Archives of General Psychiatry* 55 (1998): 1033–1044.
27. S. Wilkinson, "Aromatherapy and Massage in Palliative Care," *International Journal of Palliative Nursing* 1 (1995): 21–30.
28. Hobbs, *Stress and Natural Healing,* 188–190.
29. Newall, Anderson, and Phillipson, *Herbal Medicines,* 162–163.
30. Hobbs, *Stress and Natural Healing,* 192–194.
31. Wong, Smith, and Boon, "Herbal Remedies in Psychiatric Practice," 1033–1044.
32. M. A. Diego, N. A. Jones, R. Field, et al., "Aromatherapy Positively Affects Mood, EEG Patterns of Alertness and Math Computations," *International Journal of Neuroscience* 96 (1998): 217–224.
33. C. Dunn, J. Sleep, and D. Collett, "Sensing an Improvement: An Experimental Study to Evaluate the Use of Aromatherapy, Massage, and Periods of Rest in an Intensive Care Unit," *Journal of Advanced Nursing* 21 (1995): 34–40.
34. Hobbs, *Stress and Natural Healing,* 197–199.
35. Ibid., 200–202.
36. Newall, Anderson, and Phillipson, *Herbal Medicines,* 206–207.
37. Hobbs, *Stress and Natural Healing,* 202–203.
38. Wong, Smith, and Boon, "Herbal Remedies in Psychiatric Practice," 1033–1044.
39. P. J. Houghton, "The Scientific Basis for the Reputed Activity of Valerian," *Journal of Pharmacy and Pharmacology* 51 (1999): 505–512.
40. Hobbs, *Stress and Natural Healing,* 210–212.
41. Ibid.

CHAPTER 5

1. D. M. Eisenberg, R. B. Davis, S. L. Ettner, et al., "Trends in Alternative Medicine Use in the United States, 1990–1997," *Journal of the American Medical Association* 280 (1998): 1569–1575.
2. C. Luigi, "5300 Years Ago, the Ice Man Used Natural Laxatives and Antibiotics," *Lancet* 352 (1998): 1864.

3. D. Rennie, "Fair Conduct and Fair Reporting of Clinical Trials," *Journal of the American Medical Association* 282 (1999): 1766–1768.
4. A.-C. Nyquist, R. Gonzales, J. F. Steiner, et al., "Antibiotic Prescribing for Children with Colds, Upper Respiratory Tract Infections, and Bronchitis," *Journal of the American Medical Association* 279 (1998): 875–877.
5. B. Schwartz, A. G. Mainous, and S. M. Marcy, "Why Do Physicians Prescribe Antibiotics for Children with Upper Respiratory Tract Infections?" *Journal of the American Medical Association* 279 (1998): 881–882.
6. D. Grady, "FDA Revising Guidelines on Antibiotics for Animals," *New York Times*, 8 March 1999, www.NYTIMES.com.
7. Smith, Besser, Hedberg, et al., "Quinolone-resistant *Campylobacter jejuni* Infections," 1525–1532.

CHAPTER 6
1. Andrew Weil, *Spontaneous Healing* (New York: Knopf, 1995).
2. A. L. Wales, "The Work of William Garner Sutherland," *Journal of the American Osteopathic Association* 71 (1972): 788–793.
3. Sarah Pattee, "A Touch Opens Door to Healing," *Los Angeles Times*, San Diego County edition, 3 October 1990, sec. E.
4. D. M. Amalfitano, "The Osteopathic Thoracic-lymphatic Pump: A Review of the Historical Literature," *Journal of Osteopathic Medicine* (April–May 1987): 20–24.
5. Weil, *Spontaneous Healing*, 24–39.
6. W. J. Pintal and M. E. Kurtz, "An Integrated Osteopathic Treatment Approach in Acute Otitis Media," *Journal of the American Osteopathic Association* 89 (1989): 1139–1141.
7. I. C. Schmidt, "Osteopathic Manipulative Therapy as a Primary Factor in the Management of Upper, Middle, and Pararespiratory Infections," *Journal of the American Osteopathic Association* 81 (1982): 382–388.
8. T. W. Allen, "Coming Full Circle: Osteopathic Manipulative Treatment and Immunity," *Journal of the American Osteopathic Association* 98 (1998): 204.
9. Victor Bott, *Spiritual Science and the Art of Healing* (Rochester, Vt.: Healing Arts Press, 1996).
10. Intellihealth news www.intellihealth.com
11. The Burton Goldberg Group, *Alternative Medicine* (Fife, Wash.: Future Medicine Publishing, Inc., 1995).
12. National Institutes of Health, Consensus Statement on Acupuncture. URL odp.od.nih.gov/concensus/cons/107/107_statement.htm
13. B. Wu, "Effect of Acupuncture on the Regulation of Cell-mediated Immunity in Patients with Malignant Tumors," *Chen Tzu Yen Acupuncture Research* 20 (1995): 67–71.
14. S. J. Liao and T. A. Liao, "Acupuncture Treatment for *Herpes simplex* Infections. A Clinical Case Report," *Acupuncture and Electro-Therapeutics Research* 16 (1991): 135–142.
15. "Breastfeeding and the Use of Human Milk: Policy Statement of the American Academy of Pediatrics," *Pediatrics* 100 (1997): 1035–1039.

CHAPTER 7

1. I. B. Bassett, D. L. Pannowitz, and R. S. C. Barnetson, "A Comparative Study of Tea-Tree Oil Versus Benzoylperoxide in the Treatment of Acne," *The Medical Journal of Australia* 153 (1990): 455–458.

2. J. Lesher, N. Levine, and P. Treadwell, "Fungal Skin Infections: Common but Stubborn," *Patient Care* 28 (1994): 16–31.

3. B. G. Katzung, *Basic and Clinical Pharmacology*, 6th ed. (Norwalk, Conn.: Appleton and Lange, 1995).

4. V. M. Mahajan, A. Sharma, and A. Rattan, "Antimycotic Activity of Berberine Sulphate: An Alkaloid from an Indian Medicinal Herb," *Sabouraudia* 20 (1982): 79–81.

5. K. C. Godowski, "Antimicrobial Action of Sanguinarine," *Journal of Clinical Dentistry* 1 (1989): 96–101.

6. K. S. Nakamoto. S. Sadamori, and T. Hamada, "Effects of Crude Drugs and Berberine Hydrochloride on the Activities of Fungi," *Journal of Prosthetic Dentistry* (1990): 691–694.

7. Heneka, *"Chamomilla recutita,"* 33–39.

8. Newall, Anderson, and Phillipson, *Herbal Medicines,* 69–73.

9. P. Aertgeerts, M. Albring, F. Klaschka, et al., "Comparison of Kamillosan Cream (2 g Ethanolic Extract from Chamomile Flowers in 100 g Cream) Versus Steroidal (0.25% Hydrocortisone, 0.75% Fluocortin Butyl Ester) and Non-steroidal (5% bufexamac) Dermatics in the Maintenance Therapy of Eczema," *Zeitschrift for Hautkrankheiten* 60 (1985): 270–277.

10. K. A. Hammer, C. F. Carson, T. V. Riley, et al., "Susceptibility of Transient and Commensal Skin Flora to the Essential Oil of *Melaleuca alternifolia* (Tea Tree Oil)," *American Journal of Infection Control* 24 (1996): 186–189.

11. K. A. Hammer, C. F. Carson, and T. V. Riley, "In Vitro Susceptibility of *Malassezia furfur* to the Essential Oil of *Melaleuca alternifolia,"* *Journal of Medical Veterinary Mycology* 35 (1997): 375–377.

12. M. M. Tong, P. M. Altman, and R. S. Barnetson, "Tea Tree Oil in the Treatment of Tinea Pedis," *Australasian Journal of Dermatology* 33 (1992): 145–149.

13. D. S. Buck, D. M. Nidorf, and J. G. Addino, "Comparison of Two Topical Preparations for the Treatment of Onychomycosis: *Melaleuca alternifolia* (Tea Tree) Oil and Clotrimazol," *Journal of Family Practice* 381 (994): 601–605.

14. P. V. Venugopal and T. V. Venugopal, "Antidermatophytic Activity of Garlic *(Allium Sativum)* in Vitro," *International Journal of Dermatology* 34 (1995): 278–279.

15. R. Naganawa, N. Iwata, K. Ishikawa, et al., "Inhibition of Microbial Growth by Ajoene, a Sulfur-containing Compound Derived from Garlic," *Applied and Environmental Microbiology* 62 (1996): 4238–4242.

16. E. Ledezma, L. DeSousa, A. Jorquera, et al., "Efficacy of Ajoene, an Organosulphur Derived from Garlic, in the Short-term Therapy of Tinea Pedis," *Mycoses* 39 (1996): 393–395.

17. Newall, Anderson, and Phillipson, *Herbal Medicines,* 79.
18. J. Pepping, "Alternative Therapies: Echinacea," *American Journal of Health-System Pharmacy* 56 (1999): 121–122.
19. Newall, Anderson, and Phillipson, *Herbal Medicines,* 231–232, 229–230, 256–257.
20. Ibid., 231–232, 229–230.
21. W. J. Hueston and A. G. Mainous, "Acute Bronchitis," *American Family Physician* 57 (1998): 1270–1279.
22. K. C. Oeffinger, L. M. Snell, B. M. Foster, et al., "Treatment of Acute Bronchitis in Adults: A National Survey of Family Physicians," *Journal of Family Practice* 46 (1998): 469–476.
23. J. M. Heath and R. Mongia, "Chronic Bronchitis: Primary Care Management," *American Family Physician* 57 (1998): 2365–2373.
24. Hueston and Mainous, "Acute Bronchitis," 1270–1279.
25. Heath and Mongia, "Chronic Bronchitis," 2365–2373.
26. G. V. Doern, M. A. Pfaller, K. Kugler, et al., "Prevalence of Antimicrobial Resistance among Respiratory Tract Isolates of *Streptococcus pneumoniae* in North America: 1997 Results from the Sentry Antimicrobial Surveillance Program," *Clinical Infectious Diseases* 27 (1998): 764–770.
27. Newall, Anderson, and Phillipson, *Herbal Medicines,* 108.
28. Weiner and Weiner, *Herbs That Heal,* 144.
29. M. Reiter and W. Brandt, "Relaxant Effects on Tracheal and Ileal Smooth Muscles of the Guinea Pig," *Arzneimittel-Forschung* 35 (1985): 408–414.
30. Newall, Anderson, and Phillipson, *Herbal Medicines,* 106–107.
31. Ibid., 165.
32. Weiner and Weiner, *Herbs That Heal,* 343.
33. Newall, Anderson, and Phillipson, *Herbal Medicines,* 183–186.
34. Ibid., 210–212.
35. T. Ringbom, L. Segura, Y. Noreen, et al., "Ursolic Acid from *Plantago major,* a Selective Inhibitor of Cyclooxygenase-2 Catalyzed Prostaglandin Biosynthesis," *Journal of Natural Products* 61 (1998): 1212–1215.
36. M. Matev, I. Angelova, A. Koichev, et al., "Clinical Trial of a *Plantago major* Preparation in the Treatment of Chronic Bronchitis," *Vutreshni Bolesti* 21 (1982): 133–137.
37. Newall, Anderson, and Phillipson, *Herbal Medicines,* 256–257.
38. K. A. Hammer, C. F. Carson, and T. V. Riley, "Antimicrobial Activity of Essential Oils and Other Plant Extracts," *Journal of Applied Microbiology* 86 (1999): 985–990.
39. Newall, Anderson, and Phillipson, *Herbal Medicines,* 129–133.
40. Ibid., 28–29.
41. A. Gaudreau, E. Hill, H. H. Balfour, et al., "Phenotypic and Genotypic Characterization of Acyclovir-Resistant *Herpes simplex* Viruses from Immunocompromised Patients," *Journal of Infectious Diseases* 1781 (998): 297–303.
42. James J. Rybacki and James W. Long, *The Essential Guide to Prescription Drugs* (New York: HarperPerennial, 1998).

43. Z. Dimitrova, B. Dimov, N. Manolova, et al., "Antiherpes effect of *Melissa officinalis* L. extracts." *Acta Microbiologica Bulgarica* 29 (1993): 65–72.
44. R. H. Wolbling and K. Leonhardt, "Local Therapy of *Herpes simplex* with Dried Extract from *Melissa officinalis*," *Phytomed* 1 (1994): 25–31.
45. M. Kurokawa, K. Nagasaka, T. Hirabayasi, et al., "Efficacy of Traditional Herbal Medicines in Combination with Acyclovir Against *Herpes simplex* Virus Type 1 Infection in Vitro and in Vivo," *Antiviral Research* 27 (1995): 19–37.
46. E. K. Curtis, "In Pursuit of Palliation: Oil of Cloves in the Art of Dentistry," *Bulletin of the History of Dentistry*. 38 (1990): 9–14.
47. Newall, Anderson, and Phillipson, *Herbal Medicines,* 183–186.
48. C. W. Henderson, "Therapy (Herpes) Viracea Effective Against HSV1 and HSV2," *Herpes Viruses Weekly* (23 November 1998): 1.
49. F. Benencia and M. C. Courreges, "Antiviral Activity of Sandalwood Oil Against *Herpes simplex* Viruses-1 and -2. *Phytomedicine* 6 (1999): 119–123.
50. Intellihealth, Johns Hopkins, www.intelihealth.com
51. Pepping, "Alternative Therapies: Echinacea."
52. "Peppermint Oil and Tea Best for Nose and Stomach, Not Lungs," *Environmental Nutrition* 20 (1997): 7.
53. Weiner and Weiner, *Herbs That Heal,* 106–107.
54. Newall, Anderson, and Phillipson, *Herbal Medicines,* 106–107.
55. Ibid., 135–137.
56. Ibid., 129–133.
57. Weiner and Weiner, *Herbs That Heal,* 322–323.
58. Newall, Anderson, and Phillipson, *Herbal Medicines,* 60–61.
59. Margarita A. Kay, Healing with Plants in the American and Mexican West (Tucson: The University of Arizona Press, 1996).
60. Weiner and Weiner, *Herbs That Heal,* 243–244.
61. "Myrrh: An Ancient Salve Dampens Pain," *Science News* 20 (1996): 149.
62. X. Y. Li, "Immunomodulating Chinese Herbal Medicines," *Memorias de Instituto Oswaldo Cruz* 86s2 (1991): 159–164.
63. H. Hemila, "Vitamin C Supplementation and Common Cold Symptoms: Factors Affecting the Magnitude of the Benefit," *Medical Hypotheses* 52 (1999): 171–178.
64. "Vitamin C and Colds in People under Physical Stress," *Nutrition Research Newsletter* 15 (1996): 101–102.
65. S. Marshall, "Zinc Gluconate and the Common Cold. Review of Randomized Controlled Trials," *Canadian Family Physician* 44 (1998): 1037–1042.
66. M. L. Macknin, M. Piedmonte, C. Calendine, et al., "Zinc Gluconate Lozenges for Treating the Common Cold in Children: A Randomized Controlled Trial," *Journal of the American Medical Association* 279 (1998): 1962–1967.
67. C. Conti, A. DeMarco, P. Mastromarino, et al., "Antiviral Effect of Hyperthermic Treatment in Rhinovirus Infection," *Antimicrobial Agents and Chemotherapy* 43 (1999): 822–899.

68. Weiner and Weiner, *Herbs That Heal,* 132.
69. Hammer, Carson, and Riley, "In Vitro Susceptibility of *Malassezia furfur,*" 375–377.
70. S. Boiko, "Diapers and Diaper Rashes," *Dermatology Nursing* 9 (1997): 33–48.
71. Wormwood, *Essential Aromatherapy.*
72. Heneka, *"Chamomilla recutita,"* 33–39.
73. F. Osborne and F. Chandler, "Australian Tea Tree Oil," *Herbal Medicine* March (1998): 42–46.
74. G. T. Macfarlane and J. H. Cummings, "Probiotics and Prebiotics: Can Regulating the Activities of Intestinal Bacteria Benefit Health?" *British Medical Journal* 318 (1999): 999–1003.
75. T. Butler, J. Knight, et al., "Randomized Controlled Trial of Berberine Sulfate Therapy for Diarrhea Due to Enterotoxigenic *Escherichia coli* and *Vibrio cholerae," Journal of Infectious Diseases* 155 (1987): 979–984.
76. S. Aksit, S. Caglayan, R. Cukan, et al., "Carob Bean Juice: A Powerful Adjunct to Oral Rehydration Solution Treatment in Diarrhoea," *Paediatric and Perinatal Epidemiology* 12 (1998): 176–181.
77. S. de la Motte, S. Bose-O'Reilly, M. Heinisch, et al., "Double-blind Comparison of a Preparation of Pectin/Chamomile Extract and Placebo in Children with Diarrhea," *Arzneimittelforschung* 47 (1997): 1247–1249.
78. M. Toda, S. Okubo, R. Ohnishi, et al., "Antibacterial and Bactericidal Activities of Japanese Green Tea," *Japanese Journal of Bacteriology* 44 (1989): 669–672.
79. C. W. Henderson, "Nutritional Zinc Supplementation Reduces Infectious Disease Morbidity," *Work Disease Weekly Plus,* 28 September 1998.
80. R. A. Damoiseaux, F. A. van Balen, A. W. Hoes, T. J. Verheij, and R. A. de Melker, "Primary Care Based Randomised, Double Blind Trial of Amoxicillin Versus Placebo for Acute Otitis Media in Children Aged under 2 Years," *British Medical Journal* 320 (2000): 350–354.
81. American Association of Pediatrics HYPERLINK "http://www.aap.org" www.aap.org
82. S. F. Dowell, S. M. Marcy, W. R. Phillips, et al., "Otitis Media: Principles of Judicious Use of Antimicrobial Agents," *Pediatrics* 101 (1998): 165–172.
83. M. R. Jacobs, "Antibiotic-resistant *Streptococcus pneumoniae* in Acute Otitis Media: Overview and Update," *Pediatric Infectious Disease Journal* 17 (1998): 947–952.
84. R. Dagan, E. Leibovitz, D. Greenberg, et al., "Dynamics of Pneumococcal Nasopharyngeal Colonization During the First Days of Antibiotic Treatment in Pediatric Patients," *Pediatric Infectious Disease Journal* 17 (1998): 880–885.
85. M. M. Sloas, F. F. Barrett, P. J. Chesney, et al., "Cephalosporin Treatment Failure in Penicillin and Cephalosporin-resistant *Streptococcus pneumoniae* Meningitis," *Pediatric Infectious Disease Journal* 11 (1992): 662–666.
86. W. J. Hueston, S. Ornstein, R. G. Jenkins, et al., "Treatment of Recurrent Otitis Media after a Previous Treatment Failure: Which Antibiotics Work Best?" *Journal of Family Practice* 48 (1999): 43–46.

87. Damoiseaux, van Balen, Hoes, et al., "Primary Care Based Trial of Amoxicillin Versus Placebo," 350–354.
88. A. L. Kozyrskyj, G. E. Hildes-Ripstein, S. E. A. Longstaffe, et al., "Treatment of Acute Otitis Media with a Shortened Course of Antibiotics: A Meta-analysis," *Journal of the American Medical Association* 279 (1998): 1736–1742.
89. Dowell,. Marcy, Phillips, et al., "Otitis Media: Judicious Use of Antimicrobial Agents."
90. The American Academy of Pediatrics HYPERLINK "http://www.aap.org" www.aap.org
91. M. Uhari, et al., "Xylitol Chewing Gum in Prevention of Acute Otitis Media: Double Blind Randomized Trial," *British Medical Journal* 313 (1996): 1180–1184.
92. Dr. Duke's Phytochemical and Ethnobotanical Databases HYPERLINK "http://www.ars-grin.gov/duke/plants.html" www.arsgrin.gov/duke/plants.html
93. Newall, Anderson, and Phillipson, *Herbal Medicines*, 129–133.
94. Ibid., 250–252.
95. V. G. Cooksley, *Aromatherapy* (Englewood Cliffs, N.J.: Prentice Hall, 1996).
96. Weiner and Weiner, *Herbs That Heal*, 260–261.
97. Newall, Anderson, and Phillipson, *Herbal Medicines*, 60–61.
98. Pepping, "Alternative Therapies: Echinacea," 121–122.
99. H. Hemila, "Vitamin C Supplementation and Common Cold Symptoms."
100. A. I. Ismail and D. W. Lewis, Periodic Health Examination, 1993 Update: 3. "Periodontal Diseases: Classification, Diagnosis, Risk Factors and Prevention," *Canadian Medical Association Journal* 149 (1993): 1409–1422.
101. Jane E. Brody, "Flossing Protects Far More Than the Teeth and Gums," *New York Times*, 19 January 1999, www.NYTIMES.com.
102. Warner-Lambert Company, www.oral-care.com/listerine.shtml
103. Newall, Anderson, and Phillipson, *Herbal Medicines*, 191–192, 268–269.
104. S. Sato, N. Yoshinuma, K. Ito, et al., "The Inhibitory Effect of Funoran and Eucalyptus Extract–containing Chewing Gum on Plaque Formation," *Journal of Oral Science* 40 (1998): 115–117.
105. I. D. Mandel, "Antimicrobial Mouthrinses: Overview and Update," *Journal of the American Dental Association* 125, Suppl. 2 (1994): 2S–10S.
106. T. H. Grenby, "The Use of Sanguinarine in Mouthwashes and Toothpaste Compared with Some Other Antimicrobial Agents," *British Dental Journal* 178 (1995): 254–258.
107. T. Ooshima, T. Minami, W. Aono, et al., "Reduction of Dental Plaque Deposition in Humans by Oolong Tea Extract," *Caries Research* 28 (1994): 146–149.
108. L. E. Wolinsky, S. Mania, S. Nachnani, et al., "The Inhibiting Effect of Aqueous *Azadirachta indica* (Neem) Extract upon Bacterial Properties Influencing in Vitro Plaque Formation," *Journal of Dental Research* 75 (1996): 816–822.
109. M. I. Gazi, T. J. Davies, N. al-Bagieh, et al., "The Immediate- and Medium-term Effects of Meswak on the Composition of Mixed Saliva," *Journal of Clinical Periodontology* 19 (1992): 113–117.
110. Newall, Anderson, and Phillipson, *Herbal Medicines*, 199–200, 231–232.

111. E. D. Barnett, "Influenza Immunization for Children," *The New England Journal of Medicine* 338 (1998): 1459.
112. D. P. Calfee and F. G. Hayden, "New Approaches to Influenza Chemotherapy Neuraminidase Inhibitors," *Drugs* 56 (1998): 537–553.
113. Intellihealth and Johns Hopkins, Drug Database: www.intellihealth.com
114. Newall, Anderson, and Phillipson, *Herbal Medicines*, 104–105.
115. Z. Zakay-Rones, N. Varsano, M. Zlotnik, et al., "Inhibition of Several Strains of Influenza Virus in Vitro and Reduction of Symptoms by an Elderberry Extract (*Sambucus nigra L.*) During an Outbreak of Influenza B Panama," *Journal of Alternative and Complementary Medicine* 1 (1995): 361–369.
116. T. Utsunomiya, M. Kobayashi, R. B. Pollard, et al., "Glycyrrhizin, an Active Component of Licorice Roots, Reduces Morbidity and Mortality of Mice Infected with Lethal Doses of Influenza Virus," *Antimicrobial Agents and Chemotherapy* 41 (1997): 551–556.
117. Y. Yoshida, M. Q. Wang, J. N. Liu, et al., "Immunomodulating Activity of Chinese Medicinal Herbs and *Oldenlandia diffusa* in Particular," *International Journal of Immunopharmacology* 19 (1997): 359–370.
118. S. Donta, "Diagnosis of Lyme Disease," Medscape. www.medscape.com
119. R. Barkwell and S. Shields, "Deaths Associated with Ivermectin Treatment of Scabies," *Lancet* 349 (1997): 1144–1145.
120. Weiner and Weiner, *Herbs That Heal*, 95–96, 253.
121. Valnet, *The Practice of Aromatherapy*, 209.
122. P. Schattner, "Tiger Balm as a Treatment of Tension Headache," *Australian Family Physician* 25 (1996): 216–220.
123. Newall, Anderson, and Phillipson, *Herbal Medicines*, 151–152, 119–200, 231–232, 229–230, 256–257.
124. P. Little, I. Williamson, and G. Warner, "Open Randomised Trial of Prescribing Strategies in Managing Sore Throat," *British Medical Journal* 314 (1997): 722–727.
125. P. Little, C. Gould, I. Williamson, et al., "Reattendance and Complications in a Randomised Trial of Prescribing Strategies for Sore Throat: The Medicalising Effect of Prescribing Antibiotics," *British Medical Journal* 315 (1997): 350–352.
126. R. W. Quinn, "Comprehensive Review of Morbidity and Mortality Trends for Rheumatic Fever, Streptococcal Disease, and Scarlet Fever: The Decline of Rheumatic Fever," *Reviews of Infectious Diseases* 11 (1989): 928–953.
127. A. Dajani, K. Taubert, P. Ferrieri, et al., "Treatment of Acute Streptococcal Pharyngitis and Prevention of Rheumatic Fever: A Statement for Health Professionals," *Pediatrics* 96 (1995): 758–764.
128. Quinn, "Comprehensive Review for Rheumatic Fever, Streptococcal Ddisease, and Scarlet Fever."
129. Dajani, Taubert, Ferrieri, et al., "Treatment of Acute Streptococcal Pharyngitis and Prevention of Rheumatic Fever."
130. Ibid.
131. Ibid.
132. Newall, Anderson, and Phillipson, *Herbal Medicines*, 151–152.

133. "Myrrh: An Ancient Salve Dampens Pain," *Science News* 20 (1996): 149.

134. Hammer, Carson, and Riley, "Antimicrobial Activity of Essential Oils."

135. Newall, Anderson, and Phillipson, *Herbal Medicines*, 248.

136. C. F. Carson, K. A. Hammer, and T. V. Riley, "In-vitro Activity of the Essential Oil of *Melaleuca alternifolia* against *Streptococcus* spp.," *Journal of Antimicrobial Chemotherapy* 37 (1996): 1177–1178.

137. B. Joe and B. R. Lokesh, "Effect of Curcumin and Capsaicin on Arachidonic Acid Metabolism and Lysosomal Enzyme Secretion by Rat Peritoneal Macrophages," *Lipids* 32 (1997): 1173–1180.

138. Newall, Anderson, and Phillipson, *Herbal Medicines*, 135–137.

139. Joe and Lokesh, "Effect of Curcumin and Capsaicin on Arachidonic Acid Metabolism."

140. E. Shaffer, "Less Hype, More Hope," *Canadian Medical Association Journal* 157 (1997): 1671–1672.

141. Dore, et al., "Unexpected Antibiotic Resistance of Genotypically Identical *H. Pylori* Isolates."

142. E. M. El-Omar, K. Oien, L. S. Murray, et al., "Increased Prevalence of Precancerous Changes in Relatives of Gastric Cancer Patients: Critical Role of *H. pylori*," *Gastroenterology* 118 (2000): 22–30.

143. M. Jarosz, J. Dzieniszewski, E. Dabrowska-Ufniarz, et al., "Effects of High Dose Vitamin C Treatment of *Helicobacter pylori* Infection and Total Vitamin C Concentration in Gastric Juice," *European Journal of Cancer Prevention* 7 (1998): 449–454.

144. Y.-I. Kim and J. B. Mason, "Nutritional Chemoprevention of Gastrointestinal Cancers: A Critical Review," 54 (1996): 259–279.

145. Y. Aiba, N. Suzuki, A. M. Kabir, et al., "Lactic Acid–mediated Suppression of *Helicobacter pylori* by the Oral Administration of *Lactobacillus salivarious* as a Probiotic in a Gnotobiotic Murine Model," *American Journal of Gastroenterology* 93 (1998): 2097–2101.

146. David Hoffman, *The Herbal Handbook*, 54–57.

147. Newall, Anderson, and Phillipson, *Herbal Medicines*, 183–186.

148. E. Christensen, E. Juhl, and N. Tygstrup, "Treatment of Gastric Ulcer: The Randomized Clinical Trials from 1964 to 1974 and Their Impact," *American Journal of Gastroenterology* 69 (1978): 272–282.

149. M. E. Baker, "Licorice and Enzymes Other Than 11 Beta-hydroxysteroid Dehydrogenase: An Evolutionary Perspective," *Steroids* 59 (1994): 136–141.

150. A. Tarnawski, D. Hollander, and H. Cergely, "Cytoprotective Drugs: Focus on Essential Fatty Acids and Sucralfate," *Scandinavian Journal of Gastroenterology* S127 (1987): 39–43.

151. Newall, Anderson, and Phillipson, *Herbal Medicines*, 58–59.

152. I. Chakurski, M. Matev, G. Stefanov, et al., "Treatment of Duodenal Ulcers and Gastroduodenitis with a Herbal Combination of *Symphitum officinalis* and *Calendula officinalis* with and without Antacids," *Vutreshni Bolisti* 20 (1981): 44–47.

153. L. Cellini, E. DiCampli, M. Masulli, et al., "Inhibition of *Helicobacter pylori* by Garlic Extract *(Allium sativum)*," *FEMS Immunology and Medical Microbiology* 13 (1996): 273–277.

154. W. C. You, L. Zhang, M. H. Gail, et al., *"Helicobacter pylori* Infection, Garlic Intake, and Precancerous Lesions in a Chinese Population at Low Risk of Gastric Cancer," *International Journal of Epidemiology* 27 (1998): 941–944.
155. E. A. Bae, M. J. Han, N. J. Kim, et al., "Anti–*Helicobacter pylori* Activity of Herbal Medicines," *Biological and Pharmaceutical Bulletin* 21 (1998): 990–992.
156. James Duke, *The Green Pharmacy* (New York: St. Martin's Press, 1997).
157. S. Maity, J. R. Vedasiromoni, and D. K. Ganguly, "Role of Glutathione in the Antiulcer Effect of Hot Water Extract of Black Tea *(Camellia sinensis),"* *Japanese Journal of Pharmacology* 78 (1998): 285–292.
158. C. Kositchaiwat, S. Kositchaiwat, and J. Havanondha, *"Curcuma longa* Linn. in the Treatment of Gastric Ulcer Comparison to Liquid Antacid: A Controlled Clinical Trial," *Journal of the Medical Association of Thailand* 76 (1993): 601–605.
159. S. Mandal, D. N. Das, K. De, et al., *"Ocimum sanctum* Linn.—A Study on Gastric Ulceration and Gastric Secretion in Rats," *Indian Journal of Physiology and Pharmacology* 37 (1993): 91–92.
160. S. Kadota, P. Basnet, E. Ishii, et al., "Antibacterial Activity of Trichorabdal A from *Rabdosia trichocarpa* against *Helicobacter pylori,"* *Zentralblatt fur Bakteriologie* 286 (1997): 63–67.
161. K. Gupta, D. Scholes, and W. E. Stamm, "Increasing Prevalence of Antimicrobial Resistance among Uropathogens Causing Acute Uncomplicated Cystitis in Women," *Journal of the American Medical Association* 281 (1999): 736–738.
162. N. M. Gantz and G. A. Noskin, "Targeting the Pathogens," *Patient Care* 31 (1997): 212–220.
163. J. Avorn, M. Monane, J. H. Gurwitz, et al., "Reduction of Bacteriuria and Pyria after Ingestion of Cranberry Juice," *Journal of the American Medical Association* 271 (1994): 751–754.
164. Weiner and Weiner, *Herbs That Heal,* 78–79.
165. V. S. Barsom, A. Moosmayr, and M. Sakka, "Behandlung der Hamorrhagischen Cystitis (Harnblasenschleimhautblutungen) mit Kamillenextrakt," *Erfahrungsheilkunde* 3 (1993): 138–139 [in German].
166. G. W. Elmer, C. M. Surawicz, and L. V. McFarland, "Biotherapeutic Agents: A Neglected Modality for the Treatment and Prevention of Selected Intestinal and Vaginal Infections," *Journal of the American Medical Association* 275 (1996): 870–876.
167. Kurokawa, Nagasaka, Hirabayashi, et al., "Efficacy of Traditional Herbal Medicines in Combination with Acyclovir Against *Herpes simplex."*
168. M. Kurokawa, T. Hozumi, P. Basnet, et al., "Purification and Characterization of Eugeniin as an Antiherpesvirus Compound from *Geum japonicum* and *Syzygium aromaticum,"* *Journal of Pharmacological Experimental Therapies* 284 (1998): 728–735.
169. T. A. Yukawa, M. Kurokawa, H. Sato, et al., "Prophylactic Treatment of Cytomegalovirus Infection with Traditional Herbs," *Antiviral Research* 32 (1996): 63–70.
170. P. Tianqing, Y. Yingzhen, H. Riesemann, et al., "The Inhibitory Effect of

Astragalus membranaceus on Coxsackie B-3 virus RNA Replication," *Chinese Medical and Sciences Journal* 10 (1995): 146–150.

171. Fujihashi, Hara, Sakata, et al., "Anti-HIV Activities of Halogenated Gomisin J Derivatives."

172. H. D. Sun, S.-X. Qiu, L.-Z. Lin, et al., "Nigranoic Acid, a Triterpenoid from *Schisandra sphaerandra* That Inhibits Hiv-1 Reverse Transcriptase," *Journal of Natural Products* 59 (1996): 525–527.

173. I. T. Kusumoto, T. Nakabayashi, H. Kida, et al., "Screening of Various Plant Extracts Used in Ayurvedic Medicine for Inhibitory Effects on Human Immunodeficiency Virus Type 1 (HIV-1) Protease," *Phytotherapy Research* 9 (1995): 180–184.

174. M. Grieve, *A Modern Herbal* (New York: Harcourt, Brace and Company, 1931).

175. J. A. Karlowsky, "Bloodroot: *Sanguinaria canadensis* L.," *Canadian Pharmaceutical Journal* 124 (1991): 260–267.

176. N. A. Graham and R. F. Chandler, "Podophyllum," *Canadian Pharmaceutical Journal* 123 (1990): 330–333.

177. H. J. Glowania, C. Raulin, and M. Swoboda, "The Effect of Chamomile on Wound Healing—A Controlled Clinical Experiment Double-blind Trial," *Zeitschrift fur Hautkrankheiten* 62 (1987): 1262–1272.

178. Heneka, "Chamomilla recutita."

179. Newall, Anderson, and Phillipson, *Herbal Medicines,* 87–89.

180. Ibid., 58–59.

181. H. Grimme and M. Augustin, "Phytotherapy in Chronic Dermatoses and Wounds: What Is the Evidence?" *Forschende Komplementarmedizin* S62 (1999): 5–8.

182. T. Postmes, A. E. van den Bogaard, and M. Hazen, "Honey for Wounds, Ulcers, and Skin Graft Preservation," *Lancet* 341 (1993): 756–757.

183. J. B. Wright, K. Lam, and R. E. Burrell, "Wound Management in an Era of Increasing Bacterial Antibiotic Resistance: A Role for Topical Silver Treatment," *American Journal of Infection Control* 26 (1998): 572–577.

184. A. Spinillo, E. Capuzzo, S. Acciano, et al., "Effect of Antibiotic Use on the Prevalence of Symptomatic Vulvovaginal Candidiasis," *American Journal of Obstetrics and Gynecology* 180 (1999): 14–17.

185. J. Sobel, S. Faro, R. Force, et al., "Vulvovaginal Candidiasis: Epidemiologic, Diagnostic, and Therapeutic Considerations," *American Journal of Obstetrics and Gynecology* 178 (1998): 203–211.

186. K. Nakamoto, S. Sadamori, and T. Hamada, "Effects of Crude Drugs and Berberine Hydrochloride on the Activities of Fungi," *Journal of Prosthetic Dentistry* 64 (1990): 691–694.

187. Heneka, "Chamomilla recutita," 33–39.

188. Naganawa, Iwata, Ishikawa, et al., "Inhibition of Microbial Growth by Ajoene."

189. A. Wildfeuer and D. Mayerhofer, "The Effects of Plant Preparations on Cellular Functions in Body Defense," *Arzneimittelforschung* 44 (1994): 361–366.

190. P. Nenoff, U.-F. Haustein, and W. Brandt, "Antifungal Activity of the Essential Oil of *Melaleuca alternifolia* (Tea Tree Oil) Against Pathogenic Fungi in Vitro," *Skin Pharmacology* 9 (1996): 388–394.

191. A. L. Blackwell, "Tea Tree Oil and Anaerobic (Bacterial) Vaginosis," *Lancet* 337 (1991): 300.

192. G. W. Elmer, C. M. Surawicz, and L. V. McFarland, "Biotherapeutic Agents: A Neglected Modality for the Treatment and Prevention of Selected Intestinal and Vaginal Infections," *Journal of the American Medical Association* 275 (1996): 870–876.

193. H. L. Smith, "Recurrent Candidiasis and 'Malcarbohydrate Metabolism," *American Journal of Obstetrics and Gynecology* 179 (1998): 557.

CHAPTER 8

1. D. T. Chu, J. Lepe-Zuniga, W. L Wong, et al., "Fractionated Extract of *Astragalus membranaceus*, a Chinese Medicinal Herb, Potentiates LAK Cell Cytotoxicity Generated by a Low Dose of Recombinant Interleukin-2." *Journal of Clinical and Laboratory Immunology* 26 (1988b): 183–187.

2. M. Hirotani, Y. Zhou, H. Rui, et al., "Cycloartane Triterpene Glycosides from the Hairy Root Cultures of *Astragalus membranaceus*," *Phytochemistry* 37 (1994): 1403–1407.

3. N. A. El-Sabakhy, A. M. Asaad, R. M. Abdallah, et al., "Antimicrobial Isoflavans from *Astragalus* Species," *Phytochemistry* 36 (1994): 1387–1389.

4. Sinclair, "Chinese Herbs."

5. Y. Yoshida, M. Q. Wang, J. N. Liu, et al., "Immunomodulating Activity of Chinese Medicinal Herbs and *Oldenlandia diffusa* in Particular," *International Journal of Immunopharmacy* 19 (1997): 359–370.

6. K. S. Zhao, C. Mancini, and G. Doria, "Enhancement of the Immune Response in Mice by *Astragalus membranaceus* Extracts," *Immunopharmacology* 20 (1990): 225–234.

7. D. T. Chu, W. L. Wong, and G. M. Mavligit, "Immunotherapy with Chinese Medicinal Herbs. II. Reversal of Cyclophosphamide-induced Immune Suppression by Administration of Fractionated *Astragalus membranaceus* in Vivo," *Journal of Clinical and Laboratory Immunology* 25 (1988a): 125–129.

8. R. J. Cha, D. W. Zeng, and Q. S. Chang, "Non-surgical Treatment of Small Cell Lung Cancer with Chemo-radio-immunotherapy and Traditional Chinese Medicine," *Chung Hua Nei Ko Tsa Chih* 33 (1994): 462–466.

9. J. R. Rittenhouse, P. D. Lui, and B. H. Lau, "Chinese Medicinal Herbs Reverse Macrophage Suppression Induced by Urological Tumors," *Journal of Urology* 146 (1991): 486–490.

10. Y.-Z. Yang, P.-Y. Jin, Q. Guo, et al., "Treatment of Experimental Coxsackie B-3 Viral Myocarditis with *Astragalus membranaceus* in Mice," *Chinese Medical Journal* 103 (1990): 14–18.

11. P. Tianqing, Y. Yingzhen, H. Riesemann, et al., "The Inhibitory Effect of *Astragalus membranaceus* on Coxsackie B-3 Virus RNA Replication," *Chinese Medical Sciences Journal* 10 (1995): 146–150.

12. B. Harris and R. Lewis, "Chamomile: Part 1," *International Journal of Alternative and Complementary Medicine* (1994a): 12.
13. ———."Chamomile: Part 2." *International Journal of Alternative and Complementary Medicine* (1994b): 14.
14. Heneka. *"Chamomilla recutita,"* 33–39.
15. Newall, Anderson, and Phillipson, *Herbal Medicines,* 69–73.
16. Harris and Lewis, "Chamomile: Part 1," 12.
17. ———. "Chamomile: Part 2," 14.
18. Newall, Anderson, and Phillipson, *Herbal Medicines,* 69–73.
19. Heneka, *"Chamomilla recutita,"* 33–39.
20. Newall, Anderson, and Phillipson, *Herbal Medicines,* 69–73.
21. V. H. Wagner, et al., "Immunostimulierend Wirkende Polysaccharide (Heteroglykane) Aus Hoheren Pflanzen." *Arzneimittelforschung* 35 (1985): 1069 [in German].
22. Aertgeerts, Albring, Klaschka, et al., "Comparison of Kamillosan Cream Versus Steroidal and Non-Steroidal Dermatics."
23. Barsom, Moosmayr, and Sakka, "Behandlung der Hamorrhagischen Cystitis, 138–139."
24. Glowania, Raulin, and Swoboda, "The Effect of Chamomile on Wound Healing, 1262–1272."
25. Newall, Anderson, and Phillipson, *Herbal Medicines,* 101–103.
26. "Echinacea: A User's Guide," *Herbs for Health* (September/October 1997): 24–27.
27. Newall, Anderson, and Phillipson, *Herbal Medicines,* 101–103.
28. Pepping, "Alternative Therapies: Echinacea."
29. Christopher Hobbs, *Handmade Medicines: Simple Recipes for Herbal Health* (Loveland, Colo.: Interweave Press, 1998): 119.
30. Newall, Anderson, and Phillipson, *Herbal Medicines,* 101–103.
31. D. Melchart, "Echinacea Root Extracts for the Prevention of Upper Respiratory Tract Infections: A Double-Blind, Placebo-Controlled Randomized Trial," *Journal of the American Medical Association* 281 (1999): 688.
32. W. Grimm and H.-H. Muller, "A Randomized Controlled Trial of the Effect of Fluid Extract of *Echinacea purpurea* on the Incidence and Severity of Colds and Respiratory Infections," *American Journal of Medicine* 106 (1999): 138–143.
33. K. D. Thompson, "Antiviral Activity of Viracea Against Acyclovir Susceptible and Acyclovir Resistant Strains of *Herpes simplex* Virus." *Antiviral Research* 39 (1998): 55–61.
34. Pepping, "Alternative Therapies: Echinacea."
35. Newall, Anderson, and Phillipson, *Herbal Medicines,* 129–133.
36. Ibid.
37. M. A. Adetumbi and B. H. Lau, *"Allium sativum* (Garlic)—A Natural Antibiotic." *Medical Hypotheses* 12 (1983): 227–237.
38. Newall, Anderson, and Phillipson, *Herbal Medicines,* 129–133.
39. Venugopal and Venugopal, "Antidermatophytic Activity of Garlic in Vitro."

40. Naganawa, Iwata, Ishikawa, et al., "Inhibition of Microbial Growth by Ajoene."

41. Ledezma, DeSousa, Jorquera, et al., "Efficacy of Ajoene in the Short-term Therapy of Tinea Pedis."

42. Cellini, DiCampli, Masulli, et al., "Inhibition of *Helicobacter pylori* by Garlic Extract."

43. You, Ahang, Gail, et al., "*Helicobacter pylori* Infection, Garlic Intake, and Precancerous Lesions."

44. B. H. Lau, T. Yamasaki, and D. S. Gridley, "Garlic Compounds Modulate Macrophage and T-lymphocyte Functions," *Molecular Biotherapy* 3 (1991): 103–107.

45. D. R. Riggs, J. I. DeHaven, and D. L. Lamm, "*Allium sativum* (Garlic) Treatment for Murine Transitional Cell Carcinoma," *Cancer* 79 (1997): 1987–1994.

46. K. C. Agarwal, "Therapeutic Actions of Garlic Constituents," *Medicinal Research Reviews* 16 (1996): 111–124.

47. S. Warshafsky, R. S. Kamer, and S. L. Sivak, "Effect of Garlic on Total Serum Cholesterol: A Meta-analysis." *Annals of Internal Medicine* 119 (1993): 599–605.

48. Steven Foster, "Gilded History," *Herbs for Health*, September/October 1997.

49. Newall, Anderson, and Phillipson, *Herbal Medicines*, 151–152.

50. Bae, Han, Kim, et al., "Anti–*Helicobacter pylori* Activity of Herbal Medicines," 990–992.

51. E. J. Gentry, H. B. Jampani, A. Keshavarz-Shokri, et al., "Antitubercular Natural Products: Berberine from the Roots of Commercial *Hydrastis canadensis* Powder," *Journal of Natural Products* 61 (1998): 1187–1193.

52. J. Rehman, J. M. Dillow, S. M. Carter, et al., "Increased Production of Antigen-specific Immunoglobulins G and M Following in Vivo Treatment with the Medicinal Plants *Echinacea angustifolia* and *Hydrastis canadensis.*" *Immunology Letters* 68 (1999): 391–395.

53. Rabbani, Butler, Knight, et al., "Randomized Controlled Trial of Berberine Sulfate Therapy for Diarrhea."

54. Newall, Anderson, and Phillipson, *Herbal Medicines*, 151–152.

55. Dr. Duke's phytochemical and ethnobotanical database, www.ars-grin.gov/duke/

56. K. Yamasaki, M. Nakano, T. Kawahata, et al., "Anti-HIV-1 Activity of Herbs in Labiatae." *Biological and Pharmaceutical Bulletin* 21 (1998): 829–833.

57. Dimitrova, Dimov, Manolova, et al., "Antiherpes Effect of *Melissa officinalis* L. Extracts."

58. P. W. Peake, B. A. Pussell, M. P. Timmermans, et al., "The Inhibitory Effect of Rosmarinic Acid on Complement Involves the C5 Convertase," *International Journal of Immunopharmacology* 13 (1991): 853–857.

59. Newall, Anderson, and Phillipson, *Herbal Medicines*, 183–186.

60. F. C. Stormer, R. Reistad, and J. Alexander, "Glycyrrhizic Acid in Liquorice—Evaluation of Health Hazard," *Food and Chemical Toxicology* 31 (1993): 303–312.

61. L. A. Mitscher, Y. H. Park, D. Clark, et al., "Antimicrobial Agents from Higher Plants: Antimicrobial Isoflavanoids and Related Substances from *Glycyrrhiza glabra* L. Var. *typica.*" *Journal of Natural Products* 43 (1980): 259–269.

62. Duke, *The Green Pharmacy.*

63. T. Utsunomiya, M. Kobayashi, R. B. Pollard, et al., "Glycyrrhizin, an Active Component of Licorice Roots, Reduces Morbidity and Mortality of Mice Infected with Lethal Doses of Influenza Virus," *Antimicrobial Agents and Chemotherapy* 41 (1997): 551–556.

64. II. Sato, W. Goto, J. Yamamura, et al., "Therapeutic Basis of Glycyrrhizin on Chronic Hepatitis B," *Antiviral Research* 30 (1996): 171–177.

65. T. Utsunomiya, M. Kobayashi, D. N. Herndon, et al., "Glycyrrhizin Improves the Resistance of Thermally Injured Mice to Opportunistic Infection of *Herpes simplex* Virus Type 1." *Immunology Letters* 44 (1995): 59–66.

66. G. Lin, I. P. Nane, and T. Y. Cheng, "The Effects of Pretreatment with Glycyrrhizin and Glycyrrhetinic Acid on the Retrorsine-induced Hepatotoxicity in Rats," *Toxicon* 37 (1999): 1259–1270.

67. M. Nose, K. Terawaki, K. Oguri, et al., "Activation of Macrophages by Crude Polysaccharide Fractions Obtained from Shoots of *Glycyrrhiza glabra* and Hairy Roots of *Glycyrrhiza uralensis* in Vitro," *Biological and Pharmaceutical Bulletin* 21 (1998): 1110–1112.

68. Kh. M. Nasyrov and D. N. Lazareva, "Anti-inflammatory Activity of Glycyrrhizic Acid Derivatives." *Farmakologiia Toksikologiia* 43 (1980): 399–404.

69. Christensen, Juhl, and Tygstrup, "Treatment of Gastric Ulcer."

70. "Myrrh: An Ancient Salve Dampens Pain," *Science News* 20, 140.

71. V. E. Tyler, "Gifts of Healing . . . from Herbs of the Season," *Prevention* 50 (1998): 83.

72. "Tea Drinking and Cancer in Women," *Nutrition Research Newsletter* 15 (1996): 104; "Tea and cancer," *Nutrition Research Newsletter* 16 (1997): 19–20.

73. C. C. Chou, L. L. Lin, and K. T. Chung, "Antimicrobial Activity of Tea as Affected by the Degree of Fermentation and Manufacturing Season," *International Journal of Food Microbiology* 48 (1999): 125–130.

74. K. Mabe, M. Yamada, I. Oguni, et al., "In Vitro and in Vivo Activities of Tea Catechins Against *Helicobacter pylori.*" *Antimicrobial Agents and Chemotherapy* 43 (1999): 1788–1791.

75. A. Rasheed and M. Haider, "Antibacterial Activity of *Camellia sinensis* Extracts Against Dental Caries," *Archives of Pharmacological Research* 2 (1998): 348–352.

76. Y. Hara, "Influence of Tea Catechins on the Digestive Tract," *Journal of Cellular Biochemistry* 27S (1197): 52–58.

77. S. Okubo, T. Sasaki, Y. Hara, et al., "Bactericidal and Anti-toxin Activities of Catechin on Enterohemorrhagic *Escherichia coli*," *Kansenshogaku Zasshi* 72 (1998): 211–217.

78. T. S. Yam, J. M. Hamilton-Miller, and S. Shar, "The Effect of a Component of Tea *(Camellia sinensis)* on Methicillin Resistance, PBP2′ Synthesis, and Beta-lactamase Production in *Staphylococcus aureus,*" *Journal of Antimicrobial Chemotherapy* 42 (1998): 211–216.

79. R. Hofbauer, M. Frass, B. Gmeiner, et al., "The Green Tea Extract Epigallocatechin Gallate Is Able to Reduce Neutrophil Transmigration through Monolayers of Endothelial Cells," *Wiener linische Wochenschrift* 111 (199): 278–282.

80. E. Kaegi, "Unconventional Therapies for Cancer: 2. Green Tea," *Canadian Medical Association Journal* 158 (1998): 1033–1035.

81. Y. Sadzuka, et al., "Modulation of Cancer Chemotherapy by Green Tea," *Clinical Cancer Research* 4 (1998): 153–156.

82. K. Sai, S. Kai, T. Umemura, et al., "Protective Effects of Green Tea on Hepatotoxicity, Oxidative DNA Damage and Cell Proliferation in the Rat Liver Induced by Repeated Oral Administration of 2-nitropropane," *Food and Chemical Toxicology* 36 (1998): 1043–51.

83. H. D. Sesso, J. M. Gaziano, J. E. Buring, et al., "Coffee and Tea Intake and the Risk of Myocardial Infarction," *American Journal of Epidemiology* 149 (1999): 162–167.

84. Osborne and Chandler, "Australian Tea Tree Oil."

85. Ibid.

86. A. Seawright, "Editorial Comment," *Medical Journal of Australia* 159 (1993): 831.

87. Nenoff, Haustein, and Brandt, "Antifungal Activity of the Essential Oil of *Melaleuca alternifolia* (Tea Tree Oil)." *Skin Pharmacology* 9 (1996): 388–394.

88. C. F. Carson and T. V. Riley, "Antimicrobial Activity of the Major Components of the Essential Oil of *Melaleuca alternifolia,*" *Journal of Applied Bacteriology* 78 (1995): 264–269.

89. Tong, Altman, and Barnetson, "Tea Tree Oil in the Treatment of Tinea Pedis."

90. Bassett, Pannowitz, and Barnetson, "Tea Tree Oil Versus Benzoylperoxide in the Treatment of Acne."

91. Buck, Nidorf, and Addino, "Topical Preparations for the Treatment of Onychomycosis."

92. Blackwell, "Tea Tree Oil and Anaerobic (Bacterial) Vaginosis."

93. A. Smith-Palmer, J. Steward, and L. Fyfe, "Antimicrobial Properties of Plant Essential Oils and Essences Against Five Important Food-borne Pathogens," *Letters in Applied Microbiology* 26 (1998): 118–122.

94. "Essential Oils of Aromatherapy: For Smelling or Rubbing, not Swallowing," *Environmental Nutrition* 21 (1998): 7.

95. Wormwood, *Essential Aromatherapy.*

96. L. Veal, "The Potential Effectiveness of Essential Oils as a Treatment for Headlice, *Pediculus humanus capitis,*" *Complementary Therapies in Nursing and Midwifery* 2 (1996): 97–101.

97. Valnet, *The Practice of Aromatherapy,* 194–197, 177–179.

98. Ibid., 150–155.

FURTHER READING

Bott, Victor. *Spiritual Science and the Art of Healing.* Rochester, Vt.: Healing Arts Press, 1996.

Brooks, G. F., J. S. Butel, and S. A. Morse, eds. *Medical Microbiology,* 21st ed. Stamford, Conn.: Appleton and Lange, 1998.

Chiras, D. D. *Human Biology: Health, Homeostasis, and the Environment.* Saint Paul, Minn.: West Publishing Company, 1995.

Cooksley, V. G. *Aromatherapy.* Englewood Cliffs, N.J.: Prentice Hall, 1996.

Duesberg, Peter. *Inventing the AIDS Virus.* Washington, D.C.: Regnery Publishing, 1996; Johnson, P. Critique of *New York Review*'s Anti-Duesberg Book Review. www.livelinks.com/sumeria/aids/phil-j/nyrev.html 11-10-1998.

Hobbs, Christopher. *Handmade Medicines: Simple Recipes for Herbal Health.* Loveland, Colo.: Interweave Press, 1998.

———. *Stress and Natural Healing: Herbal Medicine and Natural Therapies for Depression, Anxiety, Insomnia, Heart Disease, and More.* Loveland, Colo.: Interweave Press/Botanica, 1997.

Hoffman, David. *The Herbal Handbook: A User's Guide to Medical Herbalism.* Rochester, Vt.: Healing Arts Press, 1988.

Katzung, B. G. *Basic and Clinical Pharmacology.* Norwalk, Conn.: Appleton and Lange, 1995.

Murray, Michael T. *The Healing Power of Herbs: The Enlightened Person's Guide to the Wonders of Medicinal Plants.* Rocklin, Calif.: Prima Publishing, 1992.

Newall, Carol A., Linda A. Anderson, and J. David Phillipson. *Herbal Medicines: A Guide for Health Care Professionals.* London: The Pharmaceutical Press, 1996.

Schmidt, M. A., L. H. Smith, and K. W. Sehnert. *Beyond Antibiotics.* Berkeley, Calif.: North Atlantic Books, 1994.

Tortora, G. J. and S. R. Grabowski. *Principles of Anatomy and Physiology,* 8th ed. New York: HarperCollins, 1996.

Valnet, Jean. *The Practice of Aromatherapy.* Rochester, Vt.: Healing Arts Press, 1990.

Weil, Andrew. *Spontaneous Healing.* New York: Knopf, 1995.

Weiner, Michael A. and Janet A. Weiner. *Herbs That Heal.* Mill Valley, Calif.: Quantum Books, 1994.

Wormwood, Susan. *Essential Aromatherapy.* San Rafael, Calif.: New World Library, 1995.

Zimmerman, B. E. and D. J. Zimmerman. *Killer Germs: Microbes and Diseases that Threaten Humanity.* Lincolnwood, Ill.: Contemporary Books, 1996.

INDEX

acacia, 156
acne, 108–9
    herbal remedies for, 109–11, 194,
        196, 200
acquired immunodeficiency syndrome
        (AIDS), 16–17, 32, 163, 164
    and scabies, 146
    and stress, 72
    vaccine, 46
acupuncture, 94, 104–5
acyclovir, 63, 121, 163, 165
adaptogens, 68, 75, 172–73
adenovirus, 45
adrenal glands, 68–69, 70, 72
Afrin, 123
agricultural revolution, 7
Allerest, 123
allergies, 33, 46, 56, 148, 180
allopathic medicine, 94
almond, 199
amantadine, 143
amoxicillin, 51, 56, 136
amphotericin B, 50, 60–61
ampicillin, 51
angelica, 120
aniseed, 106, 147, 199
anthrax, 21, 45
anthroposophical medicine, 43, 94,
        100–102
antibiotics, 46–47, 49–50. *See also*
        individual diseases and drugs
    allergies to, 56
    appropriate use of, 59–60
    history of, 47–49
    misuse of, 53–55, 87–89, 116–17,
        151
    resistance to, 50–55, 117, 135,
        160, 163
    side effects, 47, 50, 55–59, 129

and surgery, 49
    types of, 50
antibodies, 32–33
antifungal agents, 50, 60, 112. *See also*
        individual drugs and herbs
    herbal, 113–15
    side effects, 60–62
antiseptics, herbal, 66–67, 201–3.
        See also individual herbs
antiviral agents, 62. *See also* individual
        drugs and herbs
    gamma globulins, 62
    interferons, 63
    resistance to, 163
appendicitis, 90, 91
Areca catechu, 164
aromatherapy, 78–79, 197–203
arthritis, 22, 87, 145
    herbal remedies for, 179, 196
aspirin, 157, 166
asthma, 120
astralagus, 172–75
    as immune booster, 124, 125, 144
    and urinary tract infections,
        162
athlete's foot, 112–13
    herbal remedies for, 113–15, 183,
        190, 196, 210
azithromycin, 136
azoles, 50, 61

bacitracin, 50
bacteremia, 89, 91–92
barberry, 155, 156, 185
basil, 78, 66, 159, 198
bay, 66
bayberry, 132
Beaubein, Lisa, 200
benzoin, 66

diarrhea, 54, 129–30
   herbal remedies for, 186, 131–32
   probiotic treatments for, 130–31
digestive tract, 27
Dioscorides, 85, 186
diphtheria, 18
vaccine, 38, 41, 44, 45
Doctrine of Signatures, 86
Domagk, Gerhard, 48
Dossey, Larry, 74
Duesberg, Peter, 17
Duke, James, 87, 146, 159, 189
dysentery, 5, 23, 129

ear infections, 22, 132
   and antibiotics, 132–34, 135–36, 139
   herbal remedies for, 137–39, 211
   and osteopathic medicine, 98
   risk factors for, 134–35
Ebola virus, 12, 14–15
echinacea, 178–81
   and cold sores, 122
   and cold virus, 123, 180
   and ear infections, 139
   and fungal infections, 113, 114
   as immune booster, 65
   and Lyme disease, 145–46
   and skin infections, 151
   and sore throat, 154
   and upper respiratory tract, 180
   and urinary tract infections, 162
   and yeast infections, 170
eczema, 190
Ehrlich, Paul, 31, 47
elder, 144
elecampane, 118, 119, 123
encephalitis, 8, 45, 46
endocarditis, 90, 91–92
Epstein-Barr virus, 62
erythromycin, 50, 52, 109
Escherichia coli, 22, 129, 183, 186, 193
Essential Aromatherapy, 78
essential oils, 197
   as antiseptics, 201–3
   and aromatherapy, 197
   and disease, 199–201
   infused, 208

   and insect repellents, 201
   and stress, 198–99
eucalyptus
   as antiseptic, 67, 202
   and bronchitis, 117–18, 119
   and cold virus, 209
   and dandruff, 127
   and influenza, 200, 209
   and periodontal disease, 141
   and sinusitis, 149
Eugenia jambolana, 164
evening primrose oil, 127
exercise, benefits of, 73
exhaustion, 68, 71–72

fendler spurge, 166
fennel, 67, 106, 116, 211
fenugreek, 106
flaxseed oil, 127, 132
Fleming, Sir Alexander, 48–49
flesh-eating streep. *See* necrotizing fasciitis
flora, normal human, 17–18
   intestinal, 18, 19–20
   mouth, 18–19
   skin, 18
   upper respiratory tract, 18–19
   urogenital, 20
Florey, Sir Howard, 48–49
folliculitis, 21, 150
food
   and herbal medicine, 84
   pasturization of, 5
   poisoning, 202
Foster, Steven, 75, 185
frankincense, 67, 202
fructooligosaccharide, 131
Frymann, Viola, 97
Fulford, Bob, 98

Gallo, Robert, 16
gamma globulins, 62
garlic, 181–84
   as antiseptic, 202
   and bronchitis, 119–20, 182
   and cancer, 183–4
   and cold virus, 123–24, 182
   and ear infections, 137, 211
   and fungal infections, 113, 114